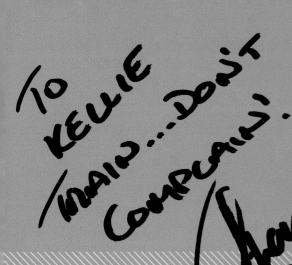
To KELLIE
TRAIN...DON'T
COMPLAIN!

Hard'n
UP Shannan
Ponton

With 20 years' experience in the fitness industry, Shannan Ponton has acquired extensive experience and knowledge in the areas of exercise, nutrition, health, people management and the media. During his career he has developed and delivered innovative personal training, fitness, motivational and general life solutions to a huge number of individuals, companies and teams at state, national and international level. Popularly known as the winning 'blue team' trainer and mentor on Channel 10's The Biggest Loser, *Shannan trains the same way he lives his life — with respect, integrity, and physical and mental discipline. This is his first book.*

I met Shannan when I was 17 years old and over the next decade had the pleasure (sometimes a lot of pain, too!) of his company both in and out of the gym. I have trained with some of the best athletes and coaches over my 25 years of training and without doubt 'Ponts' is one of the most enthusiastic, knowledgeable and inventive trainers I have come across! — *Billy Moore, North Sydney Bears; Queensland and Australian Rugby League legend*

I have known and trained with Shannan for over 14 years. In 1996, I was a 46-year-old working mother of four children, out of shape, and with a chronic neck problem. When I was 56 years old Shannan had me leg pressing 320kg (6 reps) and squatting 100kg. (No, I am not a body builder). I am now a 60-year-old grandmother and still at 61kg; I enjoy my health and fitness and apply all Shannan has taught me, training 3-4 times a week. — *Annie Richards*

I was introduced to Shannan as a cynical 50 year old with headaches, gastric reflux and hypertension, and the attitude that personal trainers were only for superstars and merchant bankers. How wrong was that! Shannan's training and philosophy has taught me that the most important measurement is not your waistline but the six inches between your ears. Once you have your brain in the right place the battle is 90 percent won. — *Dr Mike*

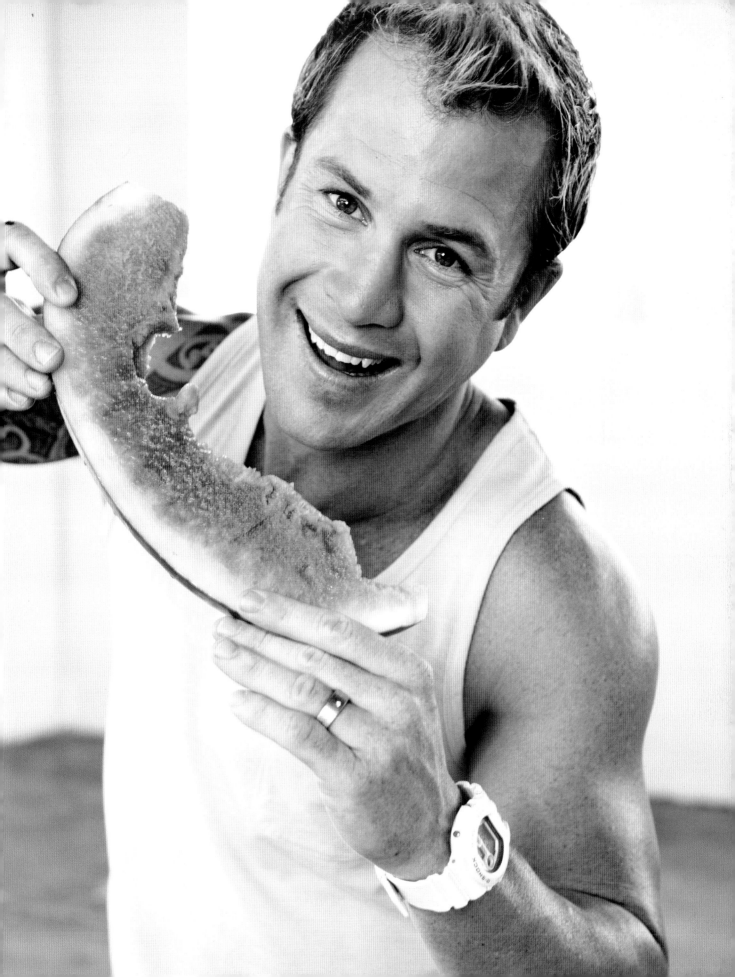

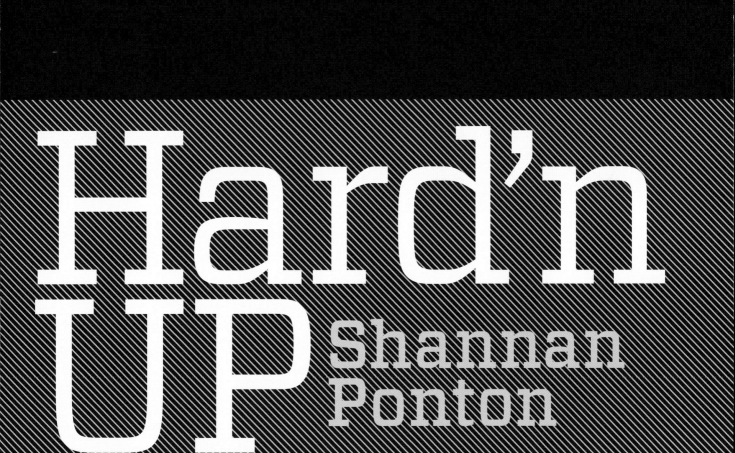

Hard'n UP

Shannan Ponton

Important information

While this book is intended as a general information resource and all care has been taken in compiling the contents, this book does not take account of individual circumstances and this book is not in any way a substitute for medical advice. To ensure safe practice, before starting any new exercise, diet or weight-loss program, please consult with a qualified medical practitioner as well as a qualified personal trainer and nutritionist or dietitian to ensure the recommendations meet your specific needs, especially if you have a pre-existing medical condition. The examples set out in this book are general guidelines and individual results and limitations will vary greatly. The author and the publisher cannot be held responsible for any claim or action that may arise from reliance on the information contained in this book.

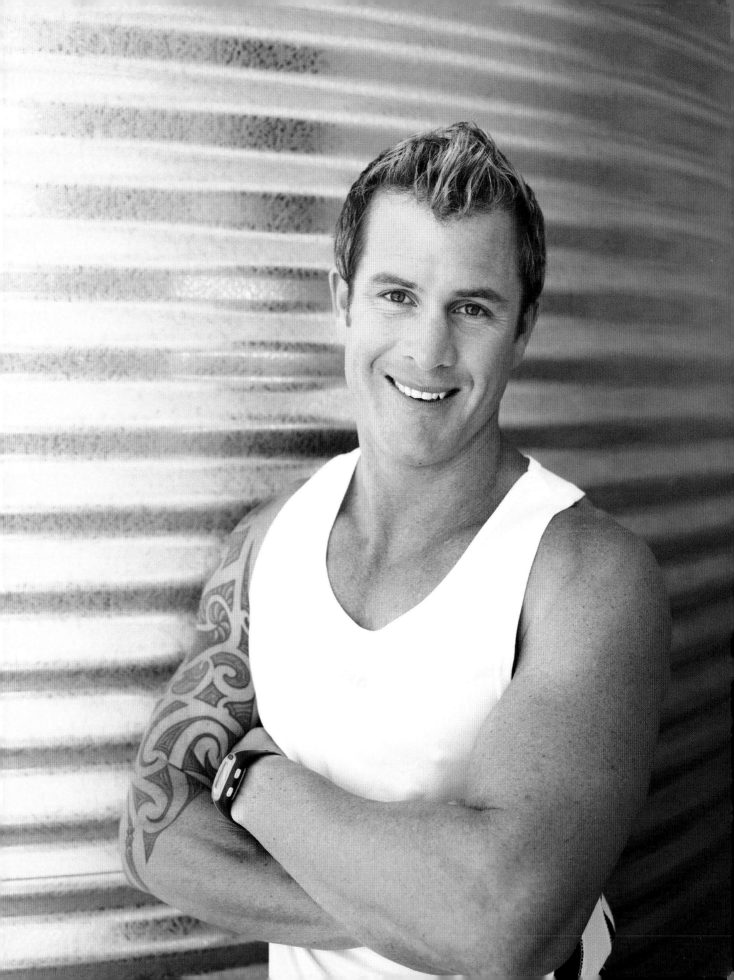

Acknowledgments   xii

Introduction: First UP!   1
• About this book   2
• Inked UP   6
• The Blue Team Philosophies   10

PART 1: PSYCH UP!   12

Chapter 1: Step UP   14
• Take control   16
• Get inspired   27

Chapter 2: Toughen UP   34
• Goal setting   35
• When the journey gets tough   44

Chapter 3: Measure UP   50
• Weigh in   51
• Assess your health and fitness   54

Chapter 4: The Heads UP   62
on Food for Fat Loss
• Eat less, move more   63
• Fess up!   65
• The big guns of nutrition   67

Chapter 5: Fuel UP —   78
The Hard'n Up Meal Plan
• About the meal plan —   80
  8 diet philosophies
• Meal plan guidelines   92

Chapter 6: Plate UP — Menu Plans   104
• Approved list of foods   105
• Menu plan for women   112
• Menu plan for men   117
• Sample menu plans   122

PART 3: SHAPE UP! — 124

Chapter 7: The Heads UP on Fitness for Fat Loss — 126
- Why exercise is king (or queen!) — 127
- Four ways to move — 130
- Top training methods — 136

Chapter 8: Rip it UP — The Hard'n Up Training Program — 146
- About the training program — 8 training philosophies — 148
- Program guidelines — 156

Chapter 9: Build UP — The Hard'n Up Toolbox — 170
- The training programs — 171
- The exercises — 192
- The stretches — 218
- Exercise outside the gym — 222

PART 4: KEEP IT UP! — 226

Chapter 10: Balance it UP — 228
- Make health and happiness a priority — 229
- Getting the balance right — 238

Chapter 11: Charge UP — 242
- Energy boosters — 244
- Jump UP for joy — 252

Chapter 12: Never, ever, EVER give UP — 254
- Keep the weight off — 257
- Tools to keep you on track — diaries, journals, logs, and planners — 262

FINAL WORD: WRAP UP — 270
- Don't sweat the small stuff — 271
- Life is not a dress rehearsal — 273

Foreword

Rewind three years. I was a completely different person; I was overweight, unhealthy, and unhappy, with no future worth living in sight. Life was passing me by and my health was slipping away.

Then I met someone who would change my bleak reality forever. From my first day in *The Biggest Loser* house I knew that Shannan would be the driving force that would turn my life around. The next few months turned out to be some of the toughest but most rewarding of my life.

After choosing Shannan as my trainer and assembling an underdog Blue Team of old and injured souls, Shannan began to work his magic, making the unthinkable happen. With Shannan's expertise, training and nutritional information, we witnessed people reduce heart problems, come off insulin, begin to believe in themselves and regain their lives.

Personally, every experience I have had with Shannan has been nothing but positive. He got my life on track. He helped me through some of the toughest times of my life, overcome some of my greatest fears, and made me the fittest and happiest I've ever been.

My biggest fear was (not heights, not spiders, not flying, and not even a training session with Shannan!) sharks! Knowing that a big part of *The Biggest Loser* experience was facing one's fears, I had no intention of sharing my fear of sharks with any of the producers or contestants in the chance I would be made to face them. On arriving at a wharf in Hawaii, I was greeted by Shannan who had a giant smile on his face. I still remember him laughing at how white I was when he revealed we would be doing a shark dive! On the 5-kilometre boat ride offshore he also told me that it was he who revealed my fear of sharks to the producers as I had apparently let it slip to him one day after a training session. That slip was the greatest mistake of my life!

I had been training with Shannan for weeks but this was going to be the biggest mental test he could throw at me. He explained that if I was able to face my biggest fear and swim with the sharks there was nothing that I wouldn't be able to do. Just 10 minutes after jumping in to the water he revealed what the real challenge was — to swim outside the shark cage! At first, I honestly thought he was kidding, but after he opened the cage I knew it was for real. I had so much trust and belief in Shannan that we both left the cage. That moment will be burned into my mind forever; it was the moment that made me realise that I would be able to win the title of *The Biggest Loser* and for that I owe him everything.

As clichéd as it sounds, a wise man by the name of Johann Gottfried Von Herder once said: 'Without inspiration the best powers of the mind remain dormant, there is a fuel in us which needs to be ignited with sparks.' Shannan was my spark, he showed me I could achieve anything.

In the first week I met Shannan, he gave me some of the best advice that I would ever receive — control the 'controllables'. He explained that there were always going to be things in life that were out of your reach and no matter how hard you try or how hard you work they will still remain out of your control. The best solution is to control what you are able to and things will generally work themselves out. There is no point wasting time and energy on things out of your control. This motto doesn't only apply to training but also to the everyday curve balls that are thrown at you in life.
— Samuel Rouen, Series 3 winner of
  The Biggest Loser

I can honestly say that my time with Shannan on *The Biggest Loser* and his continued support since has played a massive part in saving my life and giving me purpose. He will always be a big part of my past and my future. He is an inspiration and a lifesaver, but, most of all, a mate.

Acknowledgments

My entire journey would never have commenced if it wasn't for Carl and Mark Fennessey from Shine Australia, with their incredible ability to continually create cutting edge, quality TV and for the commitment and passion they have pumped into *The Biggest Loser*. I thank them also for the faith they have put in me.

I must also acknowledge the commitment, dedication and loyalty my contestants and clients have given me. Without them and their staggering, awe-inspiring, life-changing transformations there would be no book and the phenomenal results they achieve would be pipedreams and thought of as impossible. Their results should inspire our nation; after all, they're 'normal people' — if they can, you can.

My management team from Mark Morrissey & Associates, Erin and Mark, I can't thank enough. To this day we don't have any form of contract; for us a handshake is way more binding.

I've been blessed to be inspired, motivated and guided by two amazing trainers: Paul Anderson from Glovebox, is my mentor and has had a massive impact on my philosophies and methods not only for training but life; August Vaifale's skills as a boxing and conditioning coach are as good as they get. A more genuine, humble, selfless pair of trainers you couldn't hope to meet. They have both spent a lifetime in and around gyms and are still as passionate and generous with their time as the day they started.

My mother and father could not have been more positive role models. Both still regularly attend my spin and body attack classes and have lead a fit and healthy life structured around healthy eating and physical activity for my entire life. I love spending time with Mum and Dad, and I am lucky to have been shown two different styles of life. My Dad's (a proud Vietnam Vet) philosophy of 'hard but fair' seemed tough as a kid but as I matured I understood what he was getting at. My Mum is the most caring, compassionate, selfless and loyal person that I have ever met — she's one of a kind and touches the lives of everyone she meets in a positive way.

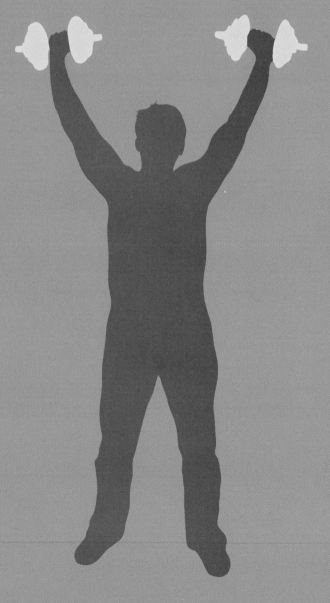

Thank you to Julian and all the crew
at Harper Collins for their guidance, trust
and understanding in helping me put
this book together, my first.

Donna Jones, my amazing writer who
managed to get into my head very early
on in this book. She has an incredible skill
of being able to express on paper exactly
how and what I was thinking and alluding
to. Donna is a world-class writer with no
less than five books under her belt. I thank
her for her patience and making the 'hard
yards' in this book enjoyable.

Final mention, appropriately, goes to my
beautiful wife Kylie who puts up with more
than anyone. Her patience and gracious
nature define her and defuse many testing
situations that present themselves in
daily life. She is the ying to my yang, the
sleep-in to my early start, the stash of
chocolate and chips to my tuna and protein
bars, but it works. I have never been more
at peace and ease, with life and myself,
since getting married. Thank you angel.

Introduction:
First UP

We're facing a scary time in society with two-thirds of adult Australians and one-quarter of children aged 5–17 years considered overweight or obese, and the incidence of lifestyle-related diseases, such as Type 2 diabetes, continuing to rise at an alarming rate.

The good news is you don't have to be one of these statistics. No matter how unfit, overweight or unhealthy you are, you can turn your weight and health around. But you need to take control. It's time for society to hard'n up and take personal responsibility for the health of the nation and our kids — starting with YOU!

The driving force in my life is the absolute passion for a fit and healthy lifestyle and I want to help pass on the benefits of this to all the people I come in contact with.

My whole life has been dedicated to health and fitness in one way or another. I played footy as a kid, but after many injuries, I was told I'd never play football again. I was devastated, but this turned out to be a blessing in disguise: it gave me an introduction to the fitness industry as I took on the role of the strength and conditioning coach for the North Sydney Bears in the National Rugby League (NRL). I started out as a carpenter but it

was the fitness industry that I was really passionate about and I ended up working full time as a coach, gym instructor, personal trainer, director of my own personal training business, and then as a trainer of the Blue Team on Network Ten's *The Biggest Loser*.

After working in the industry for more than 20 years and being part of the massive transformations that have taken place on the show, I'm still in awe of the resilience of the human body and spirit, and amazed at how much, and how quickly, the body can change with the right diet, exercise and self-belief.

I'm motivated to help people overcome adversity, face their demons, rediscover their inner fire of desire, stay the course, conquer challenges and get their best life back. Throughout this book I can help you do the same. With hard training, good nutrition and a bit of blood, sweat and tears you can radically transform your body and your life. You can do it. I believe in you.

Do the **hard** yards **'n'** move on **up!**

About this book

The fact that you've picked up this book means things are already looking UP! This is what this book is about; recognising and taking responsibility for yourself and your life, being brutally honest in identifying where you're *really* at, then doing the hard yards to pull yourself UP out of the hole you've been hiding in to a place (and body) you want to be in.

For those of you familiar with my training style from watching *The Biggest Loser*, you'd know that I'm all about tough love and I don't sugar-coat anything. This book doesn't differ from that — I'm going to tell it like it is and be hard on you!

I train the same way I live — with respect, integrity, physical and mental discipline. My training philosophy is as it is in life — hard but fair. And I want to instil these same values into the very fibre of your being and body.

Losing weight and changing the years of bad habits that have led you to be overweight, unfit and unhealthy is tough.

There is no easy way; you simply can't escape the hard yards of diet and exercise in order to get results. I may take a hard-line approach to diet and exercise but my approach works. Just look at my track record. I've had a five out of five success rate, with all of *The Biggest Loser* winners on my time on the show coming from my Blue Team: Chris Garling (Series 2 — my first season with the show) entered as an outsider from the Black Team and trained with the Blue Team when he came in; Sam Rouen (Series 3 — Blue Team); Bob Herdsman (Series 4 — originally from the Blue Team, then full credit to the Commando who took over, completing the awe-inspiring transformation for

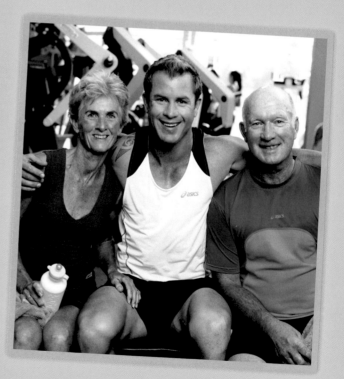

the final six weeks); Lisa Hose (Series 5 — Blue Team); biggest weight loss of the eliminated contestants, Sharlene Westren, and winning family for most combined weight loss, The Westrens (Series 6 — Blue Team).

Successful weight loss comes from consistency, discipline and self-belief. Apply these values and give them your all. You can be a weight-loss winner too.

I'm going to share with you the secrets behind the phenomenal weight-loss success you've watched on the show as well as the formula I've developed working as a personal trainer and coach for 20 years.

There are four stages to changing your life and your body. To successfully lose weight you have to:

1. Psych Up;

2. Eat Up;

3. Shape Up; and

4. Keep it Up.

In Part 1: Psych Up, I'm going to ignite that spark of motivation you will need to go the full distance of your weight-loss journey.

In Part 2: Eat Up, I'm going to reveal to you the eating plan I use with my Biggest Loser contestants, which has allowed all of them to lose masses of weight in a short amount of time.

7 tips for sure-fire weight loss

1. Get a good personal trainer, gym, and/or training partner.

2. Hard'n up, stop making excuses and just do it.

3. Be disciplined and consistent with training and nutrition.

4. Make a commitment to yourself and back it up.

5. Set challenging yet achievable short- and long-term goals.

6. Don't change your diet on the weekends.

7. Find a type of training that you enjoy.

In Part 3: Shape Up, I will give you a training program to see you through most of the year and a series of exercises that will get you looking lean and toned.

In Part 4: Keep it Up, I'm going to create the time and energy you will need to implement your training programs and follow a new lifestyle.

Throughout the book you'll also find anecdotes from me to give you a little insight into my life and beliefs, as well as from inspiring people who have won their battle with the bulge and reclaimed their lives.

Calories are used as a measurement of energy throughout this book. If you prefer to use kilojoules, simply convert calories to kilojoules by multiplying the calorie amount by 4.2 (one calorie/ cal is equivalent to 4.2 kilojoules/ kJ). For example, 100 calories equals 420 kilojoules (100 x 4.2 = 420).

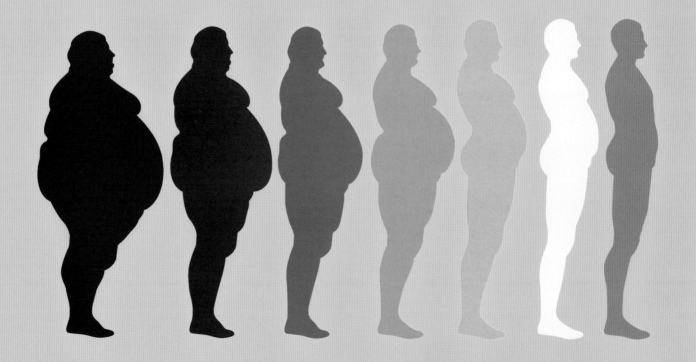

How much weight can I expect to lose and how fast?

The traditional prescription for weight loss has been a slow and gradual loss of half to 1 kilogram a week as the safest and most sustainable method. But many successful diet and weight-loss programs have been challenging this theory for years, and this line of thinking is changing.

Studies are showing the opposite to be true: that rapid weight-loss results provide people with a huge source of motivation, helping them to stick with their diet and weight-loss plan with greater ease — and it's sticking to a weight-loss plan that determines long-term weight-loss success.

People want and need fast weight loss in order to stick with the program.

Many diets fail because they don't get results fast enough. Results inspire more results.

The other argument against fast weight loss is that you're more likely to put the weight back on. On *The Biggest Loser,* we've found the relapse rate to be no different to any other weight-loss plan. The fact is people relapse and put the weight back on across all diet plans. And no matter whether you lose the weight fast or slow, with this diet or that diet, what determines whether you regain the weight or not is whether you return to your old lifestyle and eating habits.

So there's absolutely no reason why you can't lose big amounts of weight, quickly. You can lose weight as fast as your lifestyle allows. The more training you do and the better you eat, the faster your rate of weight loss.

Note: Weight loss tends to drop dramatically in the first few weeks and then slows up a little. This is normal because when you start a training program your body burns up its carbohydrate stores first, and for every gram of carbohydrate you have approximately 3 grams of water stored, so this means if you burn half a kilogram of carbohydrate stores your weight loss will most likely be 2 kilograms, taking into account the water loss (500 grams carbohydrate plus 1.5 kilograms water). But as you get further into your training your carbohydrate stores become depleted so you don't lose as much fluid. Don't be disheartened if your results on the scales never match those initial weeks, just stick with the program and, bit by bit, the weight will come off.

Inked UP

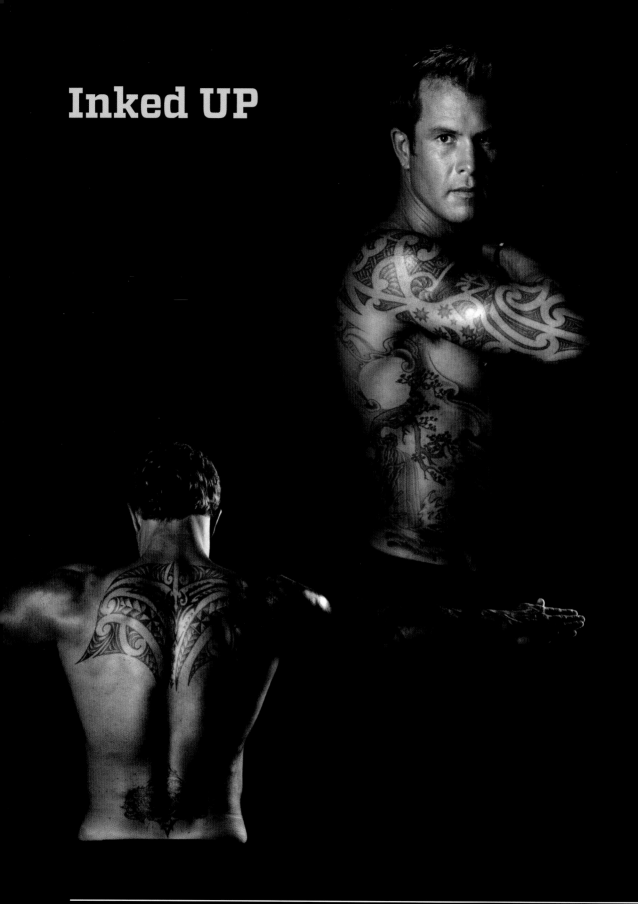

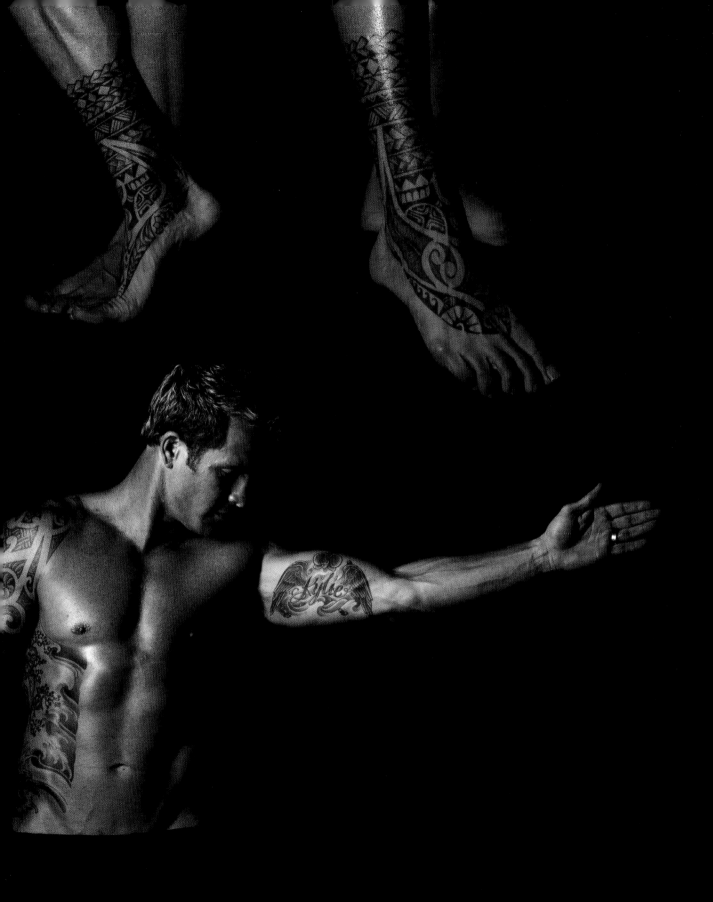

No, I'm not Maori, not even a Kiwi. For over ten years when I was a builder, the boys that worked for me were mostly Maori, in that time I fell in love with their culture. Their focus on family, respect and nature struck a chord deep inside me, something that is represented by my tattoos. The more I learned, the more I wanted to know and the boys took pride in teaching and showing me what they knew. It is with upmost respect and humbleness that I show my Maori tattoos.

The bottom part of my sleeve was done by Nathan Puata from Lighthouse Tattoo, an amazing Maori tattooist. It is called Puhoro from the Te Arawa People. It represents my life, beliefs and philosophies. The swirls represent the motion of the ocean, a never ending flow of tides and energy; what goes out comes in, what goes up must come down. The Hae Hae lines represent my family, even speaking of the miscarriages my mum had. The overriding symbolism is that all aspects of life, family, nature and self are intrinsically connected and each flows into the other.

The other parts of my sleeve were done by various artists with the two dominant parts being the cover just up under my deltoid and the symbol for family and new beginnings on the middle of my deltoid.

You can see where Nathan's work starts again and fits in over the top and runs over my shoulder, front and back, then connects up with my side piece. On the front of my shoulder is the sign for infinity (I have the same one on my foot), which symbolises the endless flow of energy — positive in, negative out — strategically placed before the negativity reaches my head. Right on top of my shoulder is a heart representing the life force or 'mana'.

On the inside of my sleeve I have the word 'respect' written in traditional Balinese, my little tribute to all those affected by the horror of the Bali bombings and terrorism in general. Also, I believe respect is the number one rule for life. Ironically, as it was being done at Demon Art in Bali, the second Bali bombing occurred mid tattoo! Luckily we weren't injured but many people were, some even killed, and Bali suffered its second major terrorist attack, something that would devastate the entire country.

My side was also done by Nathan, which shows his amazing diversity as an artist. It is a cascading Black Pine tree. This tree more than anything else in the world needs to stay grounded and never forgets where it came from (remember your roots), if it does it'll fall out and die.

It's my way of reminding myself to stay grounded. I've been blessed with some amazing fortune and opportunities but this tattoo reminds me to never get too cocky and forget where I came from. It is sitting on the side of a waterfall, one of the most powerful forces in nature, but somewhere way, way up stream it started with just a humble, inanimate drop of water. Providing that drop stays the course, doesn't get sidetracked and sticks to the destination nature had planned for it, it turns into part of that mighty force — the waterfall.

Nathan also did the piece on my left arm. Up until that point I'd always kept tattoos to my right side, I guess so I could have a 'clean side' if ever required by sponsors etc. It has my wife's name, angel wings (she IS my angel), our wedding flower and calm waters rolling below. I promised her that the left side would stay untouched now until we have kids.

The lower back has a Barong done by Made at Demon Art in Bali. It is the good god and wards off evil spirits. It represents a tenacious warrior in the battle for good to triumph over evil who can never rest as evil, even if defeated, always manages to reappear.

My upper back and right foot/ankle were done by Carl Calia from Tongan Tattoo. Like Nathan, Carl is very spiritual and has a deep understanding and connection with his heritage, each and every part of his tattoos are there for a reason.

The tattoo on the inside of my foot matches my wife's. It has the arrowhead for bravery, fish scales for safe travel over water, a flower representing new beginnings, an infinity symbol and the family weave. Across the front of my foot is a Tiki, with starfish for eyes, representing wisdom and clarity in what I see. The rest of my ankle is made up of two warrior shields and the various bands for bravery, family, dreams and the brining together and cohesion of the different dynamics of life.

Carl did a top job of converting an old tattoo on my upper back to a more Polynesian style. The top of the tattoo has the symbol for family on each side of it and flower petals as gifts. The arrow heads run out from the centre, representing bravery of a warrior; in the centre is the iron cross, which can also be seen as two birds connected for wisdom and foresight. The fish scales are for safe travel and safety in the water. The fish kissing form a figure 8 meaning eternal love.

The Blue Team Philosophies

At the beginning of every new season of *The Biggest Loser*, when I get my team, we start out by making a pledge to live by my rules of life, which have become 'The Blue Team Philosophies'. Apply these rules to your life and weight-loss journey and you will get success — guaranteed.

1. Play the game with respect and integrity — the same as in life.

2. Control 'controllables' and let variables take care of themselves. Let go of the things you can't control; take control of the things you can control.

3. Live with no regrets.

4. What goes up must come down. Don't be tricky; you can't outsmart the universal laws of life — every action has an equal and opposite reaction. If you try to take shortcuts in life, if you have improper motives, you will get stung at some point along the way.

5. Approach everything with a pure and open heart and mind; a hard but fair attitude.

With these philosophies in mind it's time to take the plunge. Are you ready to take the first steps towards reclaiming your life?

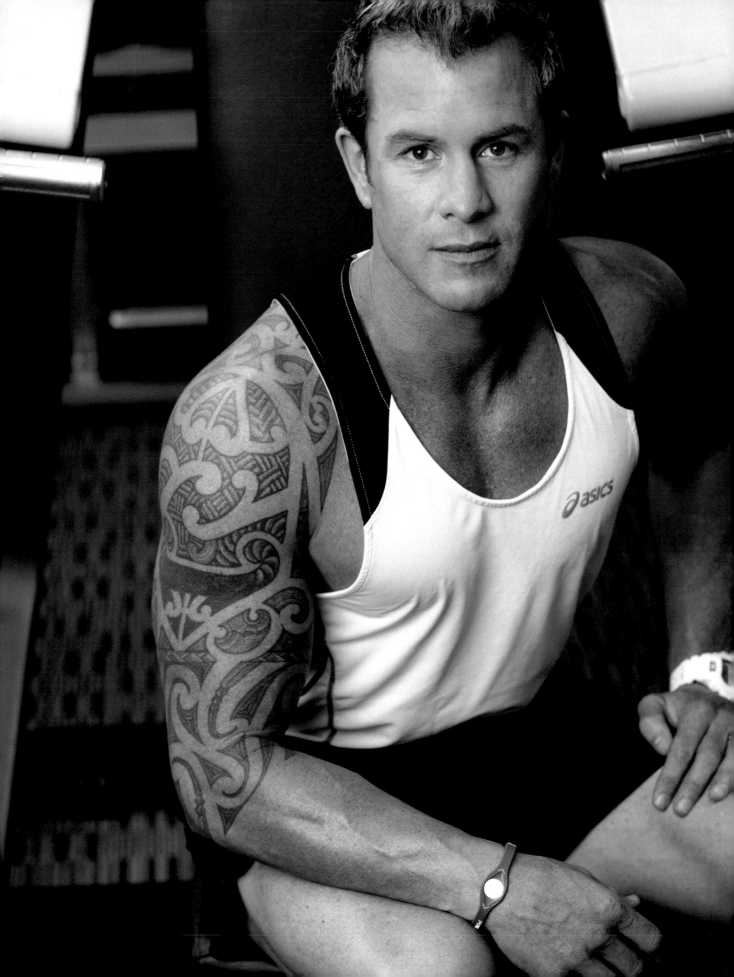

PART 1: PSYCH UP!

Do not accept anything but the very best for your body, health and life. Let's get psyched up in a big way. This is your time! No one can do it for you. Take responsibility for your weight and your life, starting NOW!

Chapter 1:
Step UP

I'm constantly amazed at the number of people who believe it's normal to be tired and less active and mobile as the years go by — because it's not! There's absolutely no reason why you can't enjoy an incredible quality of life right up until your last day on earth.

And it's never too late to turn things around. Remember Bob Herdsman, winner of Series 4 of *The Biggest Loser*? At age 56 and weighing over 160 kilograms, he went on to lose over 50 per cent of his body weight, transform his body and life, and is still living the dream to this day!

An exciting, passionate, inspired, healthy, vibrant life awaits you — you just have to step up and claim it! The first step is to understand how you arrived at this place where you're feeling broken: physically, mentally, emotionally and spiritually.

I'm a firm believer that people hold weight because they haven't dealt with the issues that turned them to food in the first place. Shannan saw straight through me from day one and my deep psychological scar (which I had buried away for ten years) came rushing out one day during training. Shannan had broken me and this release changed my life. It was like a light-bulb moment and all of a sudden I could see why I held my weight — it was my barrier, my security blanket. By not dealing with my buried pain, it ultimately led me to become miserable and overweight. From that day on, I took control and stopped being the victim. That moment changed my life. — Lara Whalan, 2011 Series of The Biggest Loser

Take control

So … you're overweight or obese, unfit, unhealthy, and possibly unhappy. Why? It's time to get brutally honest with the reasons you are the way you are, so you can put an end to the life that was, and create the life that is meant to be!

There are many factors that cause obesity and reduced physical, mental, and emotional health.

- Poor food choices:
  Society's demand for convenience has been met with an accessible abundance of fast / junk / packaged / processed foods, which all tend to be energy dense and high in fat, sugar and salt. Additionally, fruit and vegetable intake has decreased.

- Larger portion sizes:
  The size of our meals has increased across Western society, contributing to the energy imbalance of taking in more food than we burn up through physical activity.

- Using food as a drug:
  High concentrations of fat, sugar, and carbohydrates in convenience and snack foods can be addictive. These foods are being used to relieve and run from pain — depression, unhappiness, low self-worth and self-esteem.

- Lack of physical activity:
  With an increase in technology, labour-saving devices, desk-bound computer-based jobs and TV viewing time, general activity levels have plummeted.

- Social enabling:
  Society is enabling obesity. Here are some examples of how we are spoon-feeding an obese culture: fluffing and fussing around an obese person at a party, asking if they're all right, running off to get them a drink and a plate of food; making excuses, like 'Mate, he used to be quite a good athlete' or 'She's having a bad day today, she's usually up and about'; increasing chair widths to accommodate for larger people.

- Beliefs:
  'My parents were fat, that's why I'm fat,' 'It's too hard to lose weight', 'I can't lose weight', 'Healthy food is more expensive ...'. We tend to create the reality of what we believe.

- Genetics:
  To some extent, obesity is linked to the genetic material you inherit from your parents.

Just get on with it!

Being 'stressed out' is largely a state of mind. I have spoken at length with generations of my family about their life experiences. When my Great-grandfather was fighting the Germans in France during 'The Great War', I never heard my Great-grandma say she was so 'stressed out' that Pop was away fighting that she was unable to function in her day-to-day life, tend to the veggie garden and raise her kids. In her words: 'Oh son, it was tough, but we did what had to be done and just got on with it.' Think about it ... ever heard your grandparents even talk about being 'stressed out'? Be careful not to use stress as an excuse for not leading a healthy lifestyle.

- Stress:
  Modern life is leaving many people feeling frazzled and frenzied. Stress can contribute to weight gain in the following ways: 'stressed-out' people rarely follow a healthy lifestyle such as regular exercise, eating properly, or getting enough sleep; stress is a major cause of binge and comfort eating; high levels of the stress hormone cortisol are linked to abdominal fat; and when we're stressed our bodies go into famine mode (thanks to the hunter and gatherer days where food was scarce and stress was an appropriate response to urge us to go find food), making your body store fat and look for food!

Guess what? All of these factors are in your control — yes, even genetics — which means all that's standing in the way of you losing weight and being healthy is an absence of self-control.

You simply have to put an end to all of the excuses, justifications, and habits that have prevented you from losing weight. To do this, you have to take back control and break the victim mentality!

Medical causes of weight gain

Some of the medical reasons for weight gain are: an under-active thyroid, side-effects of certain medications, insulin resistance, Syndrome X and Polycystic Ovary Syndrome (PCOS). The good news is that losing weight and getting fit (working safely in conjunction with your healthcare professional) can help, even reverse, many medical conditions. Be sure to ask your doctor for alternative medications that don't have weight gain as a side effect, but be careful not to use this as an excuse — with the right nutrition, increasing your activity levels and being consistent most people will still lose weight.

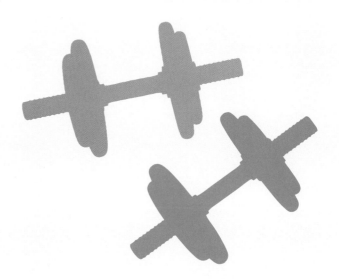

Stop the blame game

The most common factor that stops people from losing weight and changing their lives is the victim mentality, that is, it's always someone else's fault as to why you are the way you are.

People say things like: 'You wouldn't understand because … you've never been 200 kilos … you don't have a sore knee … you don't know how time consuming my kids are … my wife doesn't cook healthy meals … my boss works me into the ground and I have no time to train … you don't know how hard it is to lose weight, it's not like I haven't tried …' and on and on it goes.

Such excuses are just expressions of the victim mentality. By blaming someone else, your life situation, your environment, anything or anyone other than yourself, you fall into denial and prevent yourself from taking the responsibility you need to make changes.

If you don't eat well, it's your fault. You're the one making the poor food choices, cooking the crap, buying the junk — no one is force-feeding you! If you don't exercise, it's because you've got your priorities around the wrong way or have poor time-management skills — no one is chaining you to your desk or armchair!

When you pass the buck it may appear to be an escape from the pain and reality of owning up to your issues and your part in creating them, but it's only a temporary escape, at best — you'll never truly escape the pain you feel until you fix the problem. And playing the blame game never solved anyone's problems.

It can be tempting to fall into the victim mentality and think there's nothing good about you or your life and that everyone else is to blame. Quit it! Firstly, you can change your weight and your life. Secondly, nature tends to square everything up: where one person is lacking in one area

they are strong in another. You may be overweight but you have many great, unique qualities going for you. Change the negatives, focus on the positives and become the best person you can be.

Putting an end to excuses

Most people are armed with their list of predetermined excuses to justify their weight or lack of motivation, but the truth is I'm yet to meet anyone who cannot and does not lose weight and increase their health once they rectify their nutrition and start being more active — consistently!

Take ownership of the fact that the reason you're overweight, and possibly unhappy, is because you put yourself in this place — and only you can change it by putting an end to the excuses you make.

(If this sounds like tough love, it is! But it's necessary that you are 100 per cent honest with yourself if you're serious about change.)

Common excuse: *I'm too tired to exercise.*

Reality check: Exercise gives you energy — period.

Common excuse: *I haven't got time to make healthy meals.*

Reality check: There are plenty of fast healthy meals you can prepare in minutes, such as an egg white omelette; tuna tossed with a bag of pre-washed salad; barbecue chicken (skin taken off) with frozen vegies, steamed or microwaved.

Common excuse: *I don't have time to train.*

Reality check: Anybody can make time to train! Whether it's a walk with security guards at the crack of dawn or a world-publicised workout in a gym, most world leaders fit in some form of stress relief and exercise — and I reckon they're probably busier than most people. Whether you take 20 minutes before and after work, or cut your lunchbreak in half and train the rest or do 10 minutes three times a day, you can make a start and find time to train.

Find an excuse to train! There are no losers when it comes to exercise: it's win-win for everyone, every time!

Common excuse: *I can't afford it.*

Reality check: When it comes to food, it's usually the packaged, processed food that racks up the checkout bill, not the fresh fruit and veg, eggs, milk, meat, etc. And if you add up all of the money you spend on takeaway, eating out, coffees, and junk food, you'll soon find that you actually can afford a trolley of fresh, healthy food.

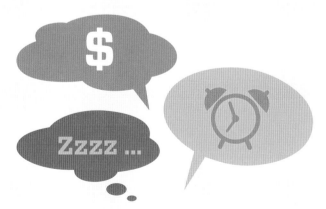

A tin of tuna in springwater costs under $2 and is the perfect eat-on-the-run, take-anywhere snack in a can!

As for exercise, walking, running, climbing stairs at your local park, doing body weight exercises like push-ups, lunges and sit-ups are all absolutely free!

Common excuse: *I have an injury.*

Reality check: I'm not saying to ignore pain or injury, but be careful not to use your ailments as a constant excuse. 'I can't do a fun run because I've got a sore knee.' What's wrong with your knee? I ask. 'Oh … it just goes,' they reply. Where does your knee go? It's attached to your thighbone by four really strong ligaments and there are many muscles that crisscross around the knee to keep it strong! 'But I've had it since high school … I just have to live with it.' No you don't just have to live with it. If there's something really wrong with your knee, fix it! If you've got a flat tyre on your car you don't drive the thing around on three tyres for the rest of your life (you're not going to get anywhere, or certainly not very fast!), you get it fixed. Do the same with your body. You might need surgery, a physiotherapist, a Pilates or pool program; rehabilitate the problem that's holding you back.

Forget the fat gene!

A big excuse that people blame their weight on is genetics — most commonly, a slow metabolism and the family fat gene. Blaming your weight on genetics is also an excuse, here's why.

'I've got a slow metabolism so I can't lose weight.'

We're all endowed with different traits: some people can remember something word for word after a single reading while others have to read the same thing 10 times to remember it. Some people are built small and some people are built big and no matter how much hard work they do, they'll never be a jockey or runway model. The same applies to our ability to maintain a healthy weight: some put on weight with the sniff of hot chips, while others can get away with eating them a few times before they put on weight (note: whether you put on weight easily or not, hot chips will eventually put the weight on you!), and, conversely, some people lose weight faster than others even though they're on the same diet and exercise plan.

Every person has a basal level of energy storage (called a metabolic set point or homeostasis). Genetics decide this. If you go over this basal level of energy storage, your body will work hard to burn off the excess energy and return itself to its set point, and weight gain won't happen. But if the energy imbalance becomes too great as a result of eating too much and exercising too little, it becomes harder and harder to return to this set point, leaving an excess of energy with nowhere to go other than — you guessed it — your fat cells!

Because everyone has a different set point of how much food and how little exercise they can 'get away with' before putting on weight it's fair to say that some people do put on, and lose, weight more easily than others.

No matter what your genetic predisposition to putting on weight, if a person is given a calorie-controlled diet and increased exercise, there is not a person who won't lose weight. We've had many a contestant on *The Biggest Loser* who'd been written off as a lost cause or thought they were not capable of losing weight because they believed they were cursed with the fat gene and a slow metabolism. Sure enough, when we got them eating less calories and healthier foods, along with exercising and upping their calorie expenditure, they lost staggering amounts of weight from the get-go.

'My parents are fat, that's why I'm fat.'

When we've had families, including parents and their children, on *The Biggest Loser* all members of the family are successful at losing weight, which totally disproves the 'family fat gene' that families tend to hang their hats on. Overweight adults blame their fat parents, then they have overweight kids who blame their weight on their parents, and so the 'family fat gene' gets passed on. But the truth of the matter is what's really being passed down through the generations is not bad genes but bad habits.

Children learn by example. 'Do as I say, not as I do' doesn't work very well — if you sit on the couch stuffing your face with potato chips while telling your child to go grab an apple, it's not going to wash. Your habits have been learned, and you need to unlearn them to prevent passing that fat torch down to your kids.

Hard'n up with your kids

Did you know that:

- An estimated 25–30 per cent of Australian children are overweight or obese?

- An estimated one in four will be obese by the time they finish high school?

- Around two-thirds of Australian families have both parents working?

- Australians have experienced a 45 per cent increase in high density living over the last 20 years?

- At least 25 per cent of Australian kids spend four hours or more per day in front of the TV?

- Heart disease is now the number one cause of death in 4–14 year olds?

- Fifty per cent of obese adolescents continue to be obese as adults?

'If you alwa

you've alwa

you'll alway

you've alwa

s do what
ys done,
s get what
s got!'

_____

It's no secret that childhood obesity is on an alarming rise. We need to tackle the problem at a grassroots level and YOU need to be a role model for your kids. By losing weight, keeping active and eating healthy, you will save your children's lives because children learn by example.

If your child is overweight, inactive and unhealthy it's your responsibility to change that. Health and fitness starts at home. Don't blame society, junk food at children's eye level at the supermarket, unsafe neighbourhoods and so on. You buy and cook their food and monitor their leisure time. You have the power to provide healthy food at home, limit TV viewing and encourage active time.

Society is now looking at taxing junk food because people can't say 'no'. What happened to parents saying 'No, you can't have that chocolate' or 'No, you can't play another video game'?

I understand that times have changed, and the days of neighbourhood cricket in the cul-de-sac have gone, but people

You can play your part in saving a whole generation of children. Lead by example and get your own weight and life under control; become a responsible parent and take the hard line with junk food, TV and sedentary time when it is needed.

When I was eight or nine years old, playing footy, everyone had these great big shoulder pads. Of course I wanted a pair like all the other kids, but Dad made me work for them. The deal: I had to make the first five tackles on the biggest bloke on the opposition team before he'd buy me some! I got the pads.

While science is discovering more and more about a person's genetic predisposition to gain weight, without a doubt, lifestyle and habits play the biggest part in weight control. So if you're not losing weight, it's because you're not eating right and/or exercising enough. Be real. Be honest. And stop blaming the fat gene!

With a genuine determination and desire to change your body and life, you can do anything. The conditions of your life are never going to be 100 per cent conducive to staying disciplined with diet and exercise — things will get in your way, such as work deadlines and family commitments — but you've just got to find your way around it, drop the excuses, stop the blame game, and get on with it! It is time to get inspired about change.

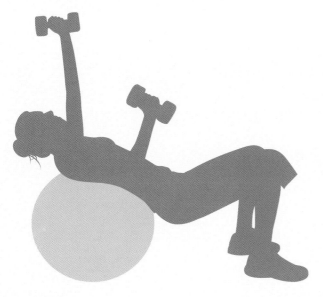

Get inspired

Health is a HUGE motivator to do something about your weight. Being overweight or obese shortens your life, is toxic to your body, damages your joints and radically reduces the quality of your life.

Obesity is associated with an increased risk of:

- heart disease, stroke, and high blood pressure;

- insulin resistance, pre-diabetes, and Type 2 diabetes;

- other diseases such as some cancers, gall bladder disease, osteoarthritis and polycystic ovarian syndrome (PCOS);

- sleep apnoea; and

- complications with fertility and pregnancy.

It's no secret then that being overweight is costing you your health and possibly your life. Don't you want to live life to the fullest and be around to watch your kids and grandkids grow up?

Heart disease is the number one cause of death in Australia, and Type 2 diabetes is increasing at an enormous rate. The chance of one of these diseases killing you is dramatically reduced if you're fit, lean and healthy. You don't get a second shot at life. The first sign of a heart attack is usually a heart attack!

The good news is, losing just 5 per cent of your body weight can drastically improve your health and lessen the scary health risks of being overweight.

What drives YOU?

To do the hard yards needed to lose weight your source of motivation has to come from a deep place within that is strong and steadfast, unwavering and constant. Sure, your doctor or family can tell you that you need to lose weight, you can read about the risks of obesity over and over, but all this will go straight in one ear and out the other or only temporarily motivate you. You need to find your *own* burning desire to do something about your weight. Let's look at what drives YOU.

There are two types of motivation: extrinsic and intrinsic.

Extrinsic motivation

Extrinsic motivation means to be motivated by a source outside of you. A common example is a girl signing up for personal training after a break-up initiated by her partner, demanding you make her a size 8, super toned and the hottest chick around to prove to the ex what he is missing out on. Another example is a guy wanting to lose weight because his partner has threatened to leave. In other words, extrinsic motivation is about doing it for someone else from a place of fear instead of doing it for yourself from a place of genuine desire to change. Kids also experience extrinsic motivation to do things, such as scoring the soccer goal or doing the sport mum or dad likes, to please their parents.

While extrinsic motivation can be very intense and powerful — just think of the lengths brides go to in order to look good in their wedding dress — it doesn't last. Take the ex-lover, threatening partner, pushy parents or wedding day out of the equation and there goes the motivation.

Without a deeper constant source of motivation that comes from within, you won't have the impetus to keep going when things get tough such as when it's the dead of winter and you've got to drag yourself out of bed at 4.30 a.m. for a cycle, when you're tired and sore and you don't know how you're going to make the last few kilometres of your run. Only intrinsic motivation will pull you through these hard times.

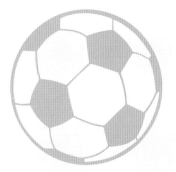

Intrinsic motivation

Intrinsic motivation comes from a source inside of you. It's the fire that burns from within. It's the sum of your passion, your desire and your commitment to achieve what it is YOU want to achieve.

This sort of motivation is essential for long-term results. It's the type of motivation that carries athletes across multiple Olympics and world championships. Look at beach volleyball player and Olympic gold medallist Natalie Cook: she's aiming to compete at her fifth Olympics. That's phenomenal! That means she's been on top of her game for 20 years. She's got nothing to prove to anyone, she's won the medals, but it's her own desire and commitment that keep her going. Another one is seven-time world champion surfer Layne Beachley — what an absolutely amazing athlete! After taking out so many world titles, she'd be forgiven for resting on her laurels. Instead, she sought out another challenge and competed in a men's surf event! Maintaining this type of motivation, dedication, and training over so many years can only come from that burning place within.

People ask me all the time what motivates me to keep being a trainer as well as keeping up my own training regime of exercising up to two hours a day, including Christmas and New Year's day, 6-7 days a week?

Helping others is a huge motivator. I've been blessed that my work has brought me success from being on the show, but that's not what keeps me going; that's not the motivation that makes me get up at 5 in the morning and give my all. It's the intrinsic motivation of knowing I'm not only making a huge difference to people's health, but also literally saving people's lives.

The other big motivating factor to stay fit and energetic is my deep desire and commitment to live a full, passionate and exciting life. To always be up for the next challenge and adventure — be it big or small.

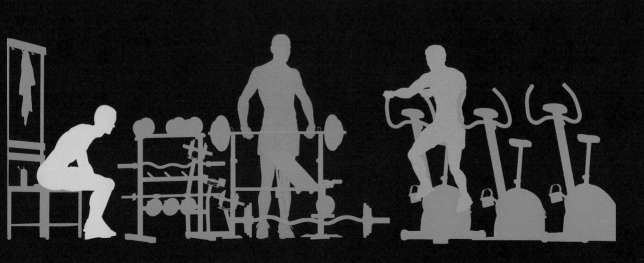

Motivation built to last

To achieve something long term, such as lasting weight loss, you need to get in touch with your intrinsic motivation.

Some examples of lasting sources of intrinsic motivation to lose weight are:

I want to feel good

If you're only trying to look good, your motivation to do so won't always last — especially if you're only trying to look good for someone else's approval, an occasion, attention or acknowledgement. If you're motivated to not only look good but feel good as well — have more energy, improve your health, sleep better and so on — eating well and exercise will become a permanent fixture in your life because the need to feel good is a strong motivator.

I want to get back some self-respect and confidence

You have to value and respect yourself in order to be successful and happy. Missing out on things — like social events, because you're too tired or self-conscious; holidays, because you're embarrassed you might not fit into the airplane seat or to don a pair of swimmers; work opportunities, because

you think you're not good enough or you don't deserve it — all diminish your self-confidence and self-esteem. And, everyday occurrences like having to get someone to tie your own shoelaces, not being able to shave your legs, or knowing that people are making snide remarks about your weight behind your back, all diminish your self-respect.

I want a better quality of life

If you're sick of sitting on the sidelines and missing out on life, you've got a huge impetus for change. To get the most out of your time on this earth and live a passionate, exciting and involved life, you need the energy, body and vitality to live it!

I want to be a positive role model for my kids

You don't want to be that parent who has to say, 'Oh, Daddy/Mummy is too tired' or 'I need a rest' or 'I can't play that game with you'. (I've come across so many overweight, unfit people who experience this as a painful reality.) When you're happy and healthy, your kids benefit by getting a parent who is fully 'there' — present and in the moment plus around to see them grow up.

My father was still playing football when I was a kid so I had health, fitness and sport drilled into me from an early age. He used to go for runs around the block, but wouldn't let me tag along until I could keep up with him. Well, I was determined to prove a point. By the age of 11 I could keep up with him, and by 12 I was kicking his ass! Both parents have set me a good example of following an active lifestyle, one they still keep up with today: they both play sport and frequent the gym (they take my spin class, which still gives me a buzz!) and my mum still has abs in her sixties!

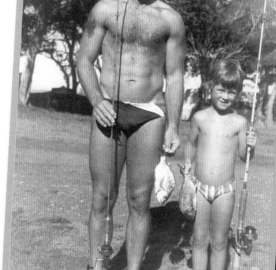

These are just some examples of types of intrinsic motivation that will motivate you for the long term.

What are some of yours? Write them here.

_____

_____

_____

_____

_____

_____

_____

_____

_____

_____

_____

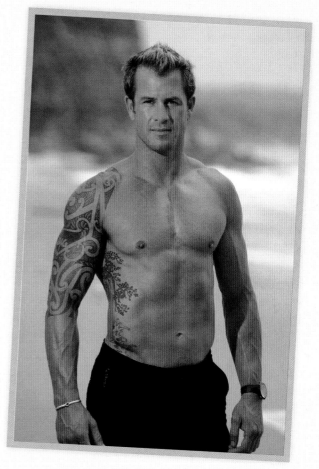

Once you find your own intrinsic reasons for losing weight, you've laid down a strong and sturdy foundation from which to build your new body and life. Think of yourself as a house, if you come against a strong wind that tries to blow you down (the obstacles you come against that try to blow you off your weight loss course), the house that is built on sand will blow down, but the house that is built on a strong foundation will endure even the toughest of conditions and stand the test of time.

Chapter 2:
Toughen UP

When it comes to losing weight it's not so much the initial impetus to get off the couch, as the motivation and mental toughness to keep going that determines weight-loss success. You've got to go from being a 'wanna' (I want to lose weight), a 'coulda' (I could go for a walk) or a 'shoulda' (I should eat better) to a doer. Do what it takes to make your dreams a reality. To do this you need to turn your dreams into concrete goals or to be more precise — your Out-of-Your-Comfort-Zone Goals.

Goal setting

Take a moment to think. When was the last time you stepped out of your comfort zone? *Really* stepped out of your comfort zone such as entered a fun run, completed a marathon, joined a gym, climbed a tree, bungee jumped, did some public speaking, karaoke, signed up for that art class, mountain biking, learned to surf, competed in a grand final, trained for a trek in Nepal, got face-to-face with lions in Africa, did that dance class with your partner. When did you last follow your hidden desires and dreams?

In series 6 of *The Biggest Loser*, Leigh Westren, who had a fear of heights, was faced with abseiling off the side of a 50-metre tall building. He froze, petrified, at the top. He couldn't get control mentally, quit and then faced the indignity of having to walk down the stairs and incur a one-hour time penalty that cost him a place in the challenge. To get over his fear of abseiling we went skydiving! Guess what? Leigh's fear of heights is conquered and he can't wait to go skydiving again. Take it to the extreme – get out of your comfort zone!

I'm always up for a challenge, looking for new ways to push myself out of my comfort zone, face my fears and live life to the fullest. I've swum with 40 Galapagos sharks (they bite!) outside of the cage off the coast of Hawaii (sharks never really bothered me until I was face-to-face with them). Despite being petrified of heights, I've skydived and bungee jumped. (I first bungee jumped in New Zealand on a series of *The Biggest Loser*. I had to put on a brave face for my team and I swear you can see my chicken legs knocking together on the footage.) I ride a skateboard, surf, mountain bike, box, run, do mixed martial arts, never giving my body and mind a chance to get stale. My mates, who are all over 35, and I are out there egging each other on to skate from the next driveway up the hill, to take on the biggest wave, to keep taking risks – I still come home with scrapes and bruises like I did when I was 10 years old. But I feel alive and excited knowing that age is no barrier.

So many people have fallen into a mundane life, where people can't identify with happiness or excitement, and can't remember what it's like to try something new. They're so content (or rather they fool themselves into thinking they're content) living in their safe bubble, just existing.

Ignorance is not bliss! Many overweight people live their life in denial as 'the happy fat person', which prevents them from doing the hard yards to reclaim their life and find true happiness.

I never want to be that bloke who wakes up on Monday morning, puts on his suit and blue tie, makes a coffee, reads his paper on the train, works all day, eats the same lunch, catches the train home, watches the evening news, barely makes the kids' bedtime, goes to sleep; gets up on Tuesday morning, puts on a grey tie and does it all again, following the same routine for the next 30 years — safe, comfortable, complacent — then retires at 55, gets a gold watch and thinks, *Wow, I'm finally here*, then dies! Now, I'm not knocking this at all. For some people this is what they genuinely desire, but for so many others they're just going through the motions, never stepping outside their comfort zone.

The same applies for exercise. Results lie outside the comfort zone. Often, overweight, unfit people will go for a walk around the block and come back and expect a pat on the back, a high-five, a 'good-on-you mate'. They think that their effort was enough. It's not! A walk around the block is way under most people's potential.

On the first day we get our contestants they train for 2 hours, solidly. They run, jump, do push-ups and they think they can't do it. But every single one of them does. And guess what? From one single session, they find a little piece of pride in themselves that's been hiding for years, and they raise their personal bar of expectation.

So when was the last time you stepped out of your comfort zone? It might be as far back as primary school. Think back to how good you felt. I want you to identify with that exhilarating feeling of achievement and accomplishment — this is how you're going to feel when you reach your goal weight and radically change your health, fitness and life!

Set yourself some Out-of-Your-Comfort-Zone Goals now and write them down here (remember these must only be goals that truly push you out of your comfort zone):

_____

_____

_____

_____

_____

_____

_____

_____

_____

Now, go back and rework these goals by:

1. Categorising them into long-, medium- and short-term goals.

2. Make sure they are:
* reasonable.
* achievable.
* specific.

For example, if one of your goals is 'I want to lose weight', you need to break it down into several reasonable, achievable, specific goals: 'I will lose 12–18 kilograms in three months (long-term goal); 6–9 kilograms in six weeks (medium-term goal); and 1–1.5 kilograms a week (short-term goal)'.

My long-term goals:

_____

_____

My medium-term goals:

_____

_____

My short-term goals:

_____

_____

Setting regular goals is a great way to keep focused and motivated through the tough times. When you achieve each goal take the time to reflect and appreciate your achievement, set yourself another challenge, and get inspired to achieve again.

Fear of failure

One of the major reasons people don't set goals outside their comfort zone is because they're too afraid of failing.

There's really no such thing as failure, providing you learn from your mistakes. Two of my favourite philosophies I love and live by are: _Only those that fail to try, truly fail at all_ and _It's only ever a mistake if you don't learn something from it._

If you have a go at something, and you _truly_ give it a go, but you fail — not because you quit or because you didn't try — simply learn what you need to from your 'failed' attempt and keep trying.

Every one is going to stub their toe in life. When you're a kid you fall over what seems like hundreds of times on the asphalt, but each time you fall, you realise that asphalt is a tad harder than skin, and you should probably pay a little more attention to where you put your feet when running, rollerblading, jumping, skating or skipping. By the time you're an adult you don't fall over anymore because you've learned through those falls (failures), how to find your balance, pay attention, focus and protect yourself.

The same is true for your goals. Each time you fall, you simply learn from it, pick yourself back up, dust yourself off, apply what you've learned and keep going until you've accomplished your goal. And in doing so, the thing you once feared is now conquered. Sometimes the falls will be small, sometimes big, but you'll find that every fall offers something positive and beneficial (providing you always see the glass as half full, not half empty) for you to implement in your learning curve, which helps you grow and evolve and move closer to achieving your goals and life's destiny.

Once you break through your fears you're left with the work of actually having to achieve your goals — which requires you to be tough.

I believe that there is a positive in just about anything and everything, but often it is unrecognisable at the time; emotion, grief and disappointment can obscure the truth.

I always wanted to be a rugby league player but I wasn't blessed with a whole heap of natural ability for the sport. But this didn't stop me. I realised at about the age of 10 that if I was super fit and super strong, I'd be able to outplay the other guys who had more raw talent than me. This is where my interest in fitness began because I realised that with training, guts and determination you could make up for a lack of natural prowess.

I trained hard, made the teams, showed a lot of promise but when I was 16 I dislocated my shoulder. I went straight in for a shoulder operation, did all of the rehab and returned to competition, thinking my life would be the same.

In the first trial of the next season my shoulder came out again. They put me back in hospital, gave me another stabilisation on the shoulder and, again, I thought life would return to normal.

During my surgery and rehab time, I took on the role of strength and conditioning coach with the

North Sydney Bears because I couldn't stand to be away from training with my mates and the sport I loved. I didn't know it at the time, but this was my introduction to a life working in fitness.

After my second shoulder operation, I rejoined the team the following season, and my shoulder came out again! After around 30 shoulder dislocations, at 19 years of age, I was told that I wouldn't be able to play rugby league again. At that time I thought it was the biggest travesty and injustice as my whole life was geared towards football. I was absolutely shattered!

Twenty years down the track and I can look at events in hindsight and with a positive mind and understand why it happened. I can see that what I thought at the time was punishment was actually one of my greatest blessings. The shoulder injury probably saved me years of bashing my body (I was also a builder by day, adding to the stress on my body). And, as I've mentioned, it gave me a start working in the fitness industry. Those words 'You can never play rugby league again' that felt like the worst failure and disappointment at the time played a huge part in where I've ended up today; doing something I not only love but also helping others.

'Don't just ⟨...⟩
the most o⟨...⟩

xist — get
t of life!'

Shannan Ponton

When the journey gets tough

You've heard the saying, 'When the going gets tough, the tough get going'. I've trained international level rugby players, kick-boxers, yacht racers, mixed martial art fighters, elite level netballers, ballet dancers, mothers, people dedicated to being fit and healthy. And the one common thread that determines success and triumph in their chosen sport and personal goals? Mental toughness.

Train your body and mind to be tough and endure pain.

We need to hard'n up! In society today, we tend to mask or skirt around facing the tough issues by self-medicating with food and other substances. But loss, pain, duress, sacrifice and hardship develops strength of character (mental toughness). By numbing ourselves we miss the opportunity to face what's really troubling us and address the pain and problems that are triggering our unhealthy and unhappy habits.

Enduring 'the grind'

The process of losing weight is tough and will involve an element of pain. But you need to work through the pain in order to gain the body and life you long for. The toughest, most painful part in this process is what I call 'the grind'.

There are three stages to any challenge be it life, relationships, training, study, sporting pursuits, or weight loss.

1. The start.

2. The middle (the grind).

3. The finish.

For example, you get a promotion with the promise of incentives and bonuses. At **the start** you're excited; you're getting more money, you feel invigorated by the change. You don't think about the extra workload, responsibilities, time away

One day I turned up to training feeling crappy and de-motivated. I had extremely tight quads, I was feeling sorry for myself, and I just wanted to leave Camp Biggest Loser and go home. I turned to Shannan before training and said, 'I've lost my mojo, please help me get fired back up'. Big mistake! Shannan took me straight into the boxing ring and started kicking me, straight into my tight, sore quads. I couldn't believe how hard the kicks were! How dare he! I thought. Shannan kept kicking me and in between kicks I was swinging punches at his head. I was furious! By the time I left the ring I was fired up all right, it did the trick. I had regained my focus and determination. Some people ask me, 'Don't you think Shannan was too tough on the Westrens?' My answer is always: 'He had to be.'

— Lara Whalan, 2011 Series of The Biggest Loser

from the family and the hard parts that come with your new job description. Then you get into **the middle (the grind)** of the challenge where things get tough. All of a sudden you're a long way from those bonuses that were promised and it becomes hard to stay focused on the task at hand. Once you get through the grind and you get closer to the target the boss has set where you know the bonus is coming, you start to come out of the grind and get a renewed sense of passion and purpose to keep going and cross the finish line. Once you reach **the finish** and you've achieved your goal all the pain is forgotten, the horrible bit in the middle (the grind) is a distant memory.

Or think of it as a marathon race. You turn up at the marathon, you get your starter pack, you're feeling great, you do your shoelaces up and they're the perfect tension, your legs are loose, the sun is out, there's a buzz of positive energy in the air and you're ready and raring to go. You think, *This is going to be the best marathon I've ever run.* The starter's gun goes off, you set out for the first 10 kilometres and you're still feeling good, then you hit the 20 kilometre mark and think, *This is great, I'm halfway there.* Things start to get harder, your legs are tired, your back's niggling and you start to doubt yourself.

At 26 kilometres, you're still 16 kilometres from the end. You're doing it tough now, things are really hurting (you're in the grind). At this stage you now need that intrinsic motivation to kick in. It's just you left to deal with your own emotions. You tough it out and start to come out the other side. Your legs are killing, but you're only 4 kilometres from the end. You can see the other runners around you, you can feel their excitement and it picks up your energy levels. All of a sudden the pain in your legs and back starts to diminish slightly; you're not so fixated on it anymore. There's 3 kilometres to go, you're so close, you look down at your watch and realise that this is going to be close to a personal best time, you've only got to run 2 kilometres and you're there. With 1 kilometre to go, the pain in your back and legs is gone, and you can see the finish line. The other runners are picking their pace up. All of a sudden you see the crowd cheering and clapping, and your energy is lifted even more. Adrenalin is pulling you towards the finish line. Somewhere you find a burst of energy and run faster to the finish. You make it! The pain is completely forgotten and you realise that all the training, the tough part of the race, the grind, was all worth it, and you start thinking about your next marathon.

Unfortunately, many people lose themselves in the grind; it's the part that breaks people. For example, in an endurance race you'll see people pull out in the dozens in the grind phase (there aren't many people who pull out at the start or when they're close to the finish line). When it comes to losing weight, anyone can start out and eat a little better, exercise a little more and lose a couple of kilos, but it's the next 5, 10, 20, 50 kilograms that sift out the people who can endure the grind.

It's in the grind where self-doubt comes in and motivation wanes, where your commitment, toughness, endurance, and staying power are tested, where every part of your mental and physical determination is called upon. This is the part of the challenge where champions are made.

Squash self-doubt and your body will respond by rising to the challenge.

What makes a champion?

All of us are created pretty equally. The human body is constructed similarly across the board. If you pinch me and I do it back, it hurts about the same. If we punch each other in the stomach, we're both going to get winded. If we get our hearts broken, we feel pain and sadness. When life doesn't work out how we've planned, we feel frustrated and disappointed.

So what sets a champion apart from the crowd? Do they have more strength in dealing with pain and discomfort? Are they better at thinking calmly and clearly under pressure? Is it that they see the positive in every situation and never give up? Is it genetic?

In sport, at an elite level, it's fair to assume that all the athletes lining up in the Olympic finals are genetically gifted and have had access to similar training — across the world, training methods don't vary that much; everyone lifts weights, runs, swims, rides, jumps, stretches, does plyometrics — but what is that one ingredient that allows one person to triumph and grab gold?

Remember Grant Hackett's incredible gold medal 1500-metre swim in the 2004 Athens Olympics? He'd been ill with a severe respiratory infection coming into the Games and people were writing him off after a sluggish swim in the heats, but in the most gruelling event of swimming, he went on to claim gold — later finding out he had competed with a partially collapsed lung. What gave him the ability to win that day against all odds? It's something to think about.

Of course you don't have to win an Olympic gold medal with a collapsed lung to call yourself a champion. There are many ways you can be a champion in your own life. Everyone is good at something. Everyone has a talent. You might just be barking up the wrong tree. What if Tiger Woods had picked up a boxing glove as a tiny tot, instead of a golf club? What if Kelly Slater decided to play basketball? We may have missed out on two of the world's greatest all-time champions.

You can be a champion at something, too. It doesn't matter whether it's knitting, a spelling bee, a seniors' race, sport, volunteering, being a master chef for your family. It can be anything. Some people are fantastic athletes, some are smart, some are creative. Do the best with the hand you've been dealt. Find the champion within you.

Champions are made of the right stuff. They have the perfect mix of key attributes — courage, determination, self-belief, desire, passion, toughness, resilience and killer attitudes. These are the attributes you're going to need to be the champion of your own weight loss. And we're going to kick off with the champion attribute you need in order to face the truth about your weight and current state of health: courage.

It takes courage to pop your head up into the light and climb out of the dark hole you've been hiding in.

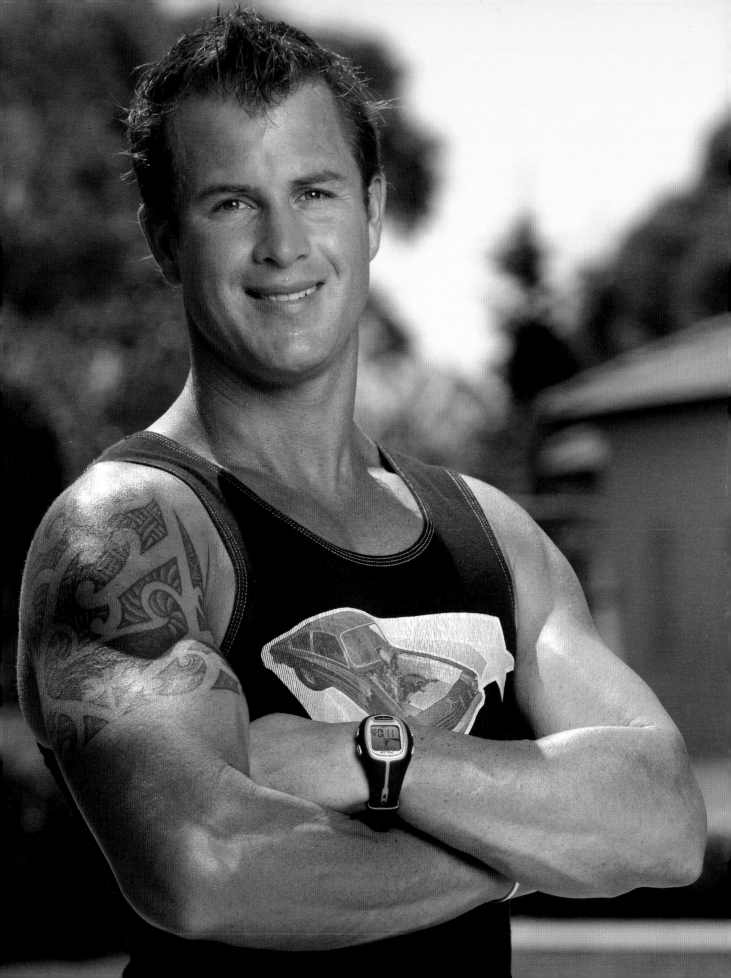

Chapter 3:
Measure UP

Before you get stuck into the nuts and bolts of the program, you need to get honest and accountable about where you're at by measuring your weight, fat and fitness levels. One of the first and hardest things the contestants on *The Biggest Loser* have to do is take off their shirts for all to see and stand on the scales. This takes a lot of courage. People often view this as humiliation, but I see it as the ultimate act of empowerment for these contestants who have hidden themselves away from the world for years. It's the first courageous step for them to reclaim their lives. Now it's time for your moment of truth. Let's see how you measure up.

Weigh in

Measurements aren't open to perception or emotion: 1 centimetre is 1 centimetre, 1 kilogram is 1 kilogram. You'll often hear people say they've put on muscle and that's why the scales are reading heavier — don't kid yourself. Yes, muscle does weigh more than fat, but it's very hard to put on sizeable muscle tissue that will show up on the scales, especially for women. If the number on the scales goes up, it's more likely that you're not sticking with the program, you haven't exercised enough,

you haven't eaten right or a combination of all three. It's also the classic 'get out of jail free' card for personal trainers: 'Oh, you're putting on muscle that's why your weight has increased'. Unless you have a specific training goal to increase muscle bulk, your weight should not increase and if it has, your trainer is not doing their job. You are the customer and you should be getting the desired results you ordered.

The best way of measuring your weight loss is by weight and waist.

Weight

Set yourself a weekly weigh-in date, *Biggest Loser* style! Make it the same time every week under consistent circumstances, that is, the same time of the day, wear the same clothes, note whether you had shoes on or off. Stand on the scales and record your moment of truth! Acknowledge where you're at and be proud that you're taking the next step.

If you're struggling to be consistent with your program, as many people do, weigh in every day. This helps ensure you don't have three or four bad (missed training sessions and inappropriate diet) days in a row by keeping you honest and accountable.

Waist

Carrying excess fat around your midsection means you're likely to have fat deposits surrounding your vital organs, which means you're more likely to develop an obesity-related illness, such as heart disease and Type 2 diabetes. Excessive waist measurements are a direct indicator for early death — it's that serious!

- A waist measurement of 80 centimetres or more in women and 94 centimetres or more in men is associated with an increased risk of obesity-related disease

- A waist measurement of 88 centimetres or more in women and 102 centimetres or more in men is associated with a substantially increased risk of obesity-related disease

To measure your waist circumference, use a measuring tape (the kind you use for sewing) and take your waist measurement.

- Wrap the tape in line with your belly button around your midsection, ensuring the tape stays horizontal.

- Don't breathe in or suck your stomach in. Breathe normally and measure on the out breath.

- Make sure the tape is snug but not tight.

Additional measurements

If you like, there are extra measurements you can do to track your weight loss and changes in your body composition.

Body fat

Measuring the amount of body fat you have in your body can be a useful health tool, because the amount of fat (as opposed to muscle) you have determines your risk of disease.

	Men	Women
Lean	<12.0%	<17%
Acceptable	12.0-18.0%	17.0-26%
Moderately overweight	18.0-24%	26.0-30.0%
Overweight	>24.0%	>30.0%

BMI

Your Body Mass Index (BMI) is used as a general indicator of overweight and obesity levels. However, it's far from foolproof as it doesn't take into account body fat distribution around the body or lean muscle mass. For example, a shorter person with a dense muscle mass and low body fat can score a high BMI, which would not be an accurate measure of healthy body fat levels; a tall thin person with a lot of muscle wastage and high body fat could score a low BMI, which also would not be an accurate measure of healthy body fat levels.

- A BMI of less than 18.5 is considered underweight.
- A BMI of between 18.5–24.9 is considered a healthy weight.
- A BMI of more than 25 is considered overweight or pre-obese.
- A BMI of more than 30 is considered obese.
- A BMI of more than 40 is considered morbidly obese.

To work out your BMI, simply divide your weight in kilograms by your height in metres squared. For example, if you weigh 100 kilograms and are 180 centimetres tall, you divide your weight (100) by your height in metres squared (1.8 x 1.8 = 3.24). So, 100 divided by 3.24 gives you a BMI of 30.9, which would put you in the obese category.

Body fat scales, that pass a safe electrical current through your body and calculate how much fat you have, are not always accurate, as fluid levels can easily skew the readings. If you are interested in measuring body fat levels, get a trained professional to use skin callipers (a special handheld device that pinches and separates fat from muscle on different sites of your body) to take your skinfold measurements, as these are much more accurate.

Girth measurements

You can also use a tape measure to measure different sites on your body. The most common ones are chest (nipple line), arms (midpoint around your upper arm), hips/buttocks (the widest point, when you view from the side), mid thigh (measured with knee flexed at 90 degrees, halfway between your knee cap and the crease at your hip), and lower leg (widest part of your calf).

Photograph

A picture never lies! Overweight people usually avoid getting their photo taken, but before-and-after photos taken on your journey can be incredibly powerful. Get someone to take a photo of yourself wearing fitted clothing — front on and side on. Notice the difference when you re-take these pictures!

Assess your health and fitness

There are some tests you can do to assess your current level of health and fitness, and, more importantly, use as a measure to see how much your health, fitness and strength levels are improving once you start a regular exercise program.

Health assessments

There are many tests that assess your state of health that you can monitor with your doctor or health practitioner, such as your cholesterol and blood sugar levels. The good news is losing weight and getting fit can manage, even reverse, many health ailments such as high cholesterol and hypertension — you may even be able to go off certain medications (do not stop taking medication without consulting your doctor).

Two simple health checks you can do yourself are your resting heart rate and blood pressure.

Resting heart rate

The more times your heart has to beat to pump blood around the body per minute, the more wear-and-tear on your ticker over time. Cardio training reduces your resting heart rate so your heart doesn't have to work as hard at rest.

The best time to take your resting heart rate (RHR) is when you first wake up in the morning. To take your pulse, sit down and place your first and second fingers on your carotid artery (underneath your chin on the side of your neck) or on the flipside of your wrist. Using a stopwatch or clock to time, measure the number of times you feel it beat in 60 seconds.

Beats per minute (bpm)	
Unfit	> 86 bpm
Average	75-85 bpm
Fit	65-75 bpm
Very fit	55-64 bpm
Elite	45-55 bpm

Normal to high blood pressure is generally between 120/80 and 140/90. The ideal blood pressure measurement is generally <120/80.

Fitness assessments

The most common fitness tests measure stamina (cardio fitness) and strength.

Blood pressure

Blood pressure is the driving force that moves the blood through the circulatory system. High blood pressure (hypertension) — equal to or higher than 140/90 — is when the pressure exerted by the blood as it's pumped through the arteries is high. High blood pressure increases the risk of heart attack, stroke and kidney failure. Hypertension is effectively reduced through regular physical activity.

Electronic machines that can be purchased from the pharmacy mean people can monitor their blood pressure at home, but you can easily get your blood pressure taken through your doctor or as part of your fitness assessment when you sign up with a gym or personal trainer.

Stamina

Cardio fitness can be measured in a number of ways, such as charting your heart rate response after walking 1 kilometre or doing a set run or bike ride, or measuring oxygen consumption (VO_2 max), which simply means the amount of oxygen consumed as you exercise.

You don't have to get too technical; the easiest way is to do a cardio exercise for a set distance or amount of time, and measure how long it takes or distance reached. You can also chart your heart rate response by seeing how high your heart rate goes from doing an activity and how quickly it returns back to normal — the faster it drops back down, the fitter you are!

1 kilometre walk/run

Find a 1 kilometre course that cannot be altered (so that the distance won't be different when you re-test). For example, on a treadmill, doing two-and-a-half laps (one lap is 400 metres) around an oval or running track, on a set walking path with measured signposts, or alongside the road after measuring 1 kilometres in your car. Walk, run or do a combination of both to get to the end as fast as you can. Record the time it takes and then take your heart rate immediately after finishing (with a heart rate monitor or by taking your pulse), and then 90 seconds later. Record the difference between both heart rate readings, for example if your heart rate was 180 bpm on finishing and 150 bpm 90 seconds later, the difference is a 30 bpm drop in 90 seconds.

Compare against your results when you re-test, aiming to reduce the time it takes to complete 1km as well as improving your heart rate recovery — improving on the number of beats it drops in 90 seconds.

Beep test

This test, also known as the multi-stage test or 20 metre shuttle run test, has been around for years and is commonly used as a measure of fitness in personal training and sports, and for fitness testing in the police force and armed forces. It's an oldie but a goodie!

To do the test you do shuttle runs between two markers, 20 metres apart, making sure you complete one shuttle run before the beeper goes off. The beeps get closer together so you have to go faster and faster to keep up. Once you can no longer keep up with the pace of the beeps, the test is finished. The stage you exit at is your fitness level. There are 21 levels (21 being the highest level of fitness reached) and the levels can be converted to give you an equivalent of what your VO_2 max would most likely be. You can access one of these tests through a trainer, purchase it on CD or download as an iPhone application, which you play through a stereo of some sort as you do the test (the narrator explains the test protocol).

	Men	Women
Excellent	>13	>12
Very good	11–13	10–12
Good	9–11	8–10
Average	7–9	6–8
Poor	5–7	4–6
Very poor	<5	<4

60-second push-up test

Do as many push-ups as you can in 60 seconds. Make sure you complete a full push-up each time with proper technique. To do a full push-up, place hands and toes on the ground. Keep feet together, body straight, hands under shoulders. Lower your chest close to the floor then push back up. Or, do a modified version by placing your knees on the ground. A description of both types of push-up is on page 194.

Strength/strength endurance

True strength tests measure the maximum amount of weight you can lift for one repetition (1 rep max), but these are potentially dangerous and need to be done under strict professional supervision. Instead, there are some great strength endurance tests you can do on your own.

	Men	Women
Excellent	>40	>30
Good	20–39	10–29
Average	0–19	0–9

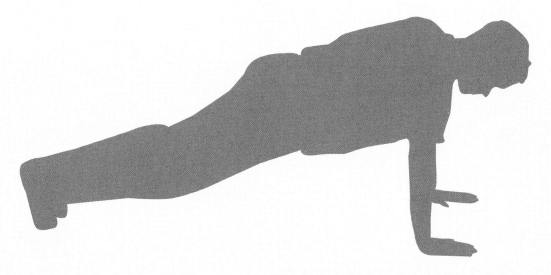

60-second sit-up test

Do as many crunches in 60 seconds as possible. Make sure you maintain proper form and complete a full sit-up each time. To do a sit-up lie on the ground with feet flat and anchored (get a partner to hold them down or hook your feet underneath something), knees bent. Fold your arms across your chest, use your stomach muscles to bring your torso off the ground, crunch up until both elbows touch your thighs. See page 213 for how to do a sit-up/ crunch.

Age	<29	30-39	40-59
Excellent	>40	>35	>30
Good	25-40	20-35	15-30
Average	<25	<20	<15

Wall squat

This is a great test for measuring strength endurance in your legs. Position yourself in a squat with hips and knees bent at right angles, back pressed up against the wall. Hold for as long as you can. Aim to hold for longer each time you re-test.

Plank

This exercise tests your stomach stamina. Prop yourself up on your on toes and elbows, feet together and elbows under the shoulders. Keep your body in a straight line, squeeze your abdominals and hold for as long as you can. Keep breathing throughout; don't let your shoulders hunch or your backside drift up in the air. See page 216 for the technique on how to do a plank. Aim to hold for longer each time you re-test and beat your personal best score.

Measure up — your results

Write your starting weight and health and fitness status on the chart on the next page, so you can come back to it at a later date and see how far you've come.

Remember, results inspire results. So take these measures again regularly, say every 4–6 weeks, to get a little boost from how far you're progressing. Simply make a copy of this blank table and re-use every time you reassess.

Now that you've gotten real about where you're at, it's time to move forwards and focus on where you're heading — Up!

Your results

Date												
Weight												
Starting weight												
Waist measurement												
Other measurements												
Health												
Resting heart rate												
Blood pressure												
Other health results												
Fitness												
1 kilometre walk/ run: Time												
Heart rate												
Beep test: Level reached												
60-second push-up test: How many												
60-second sit-up test: How many												
Wall squat: How long												
Plank: How long												
Any additional tests												

MEASURE UP

PART 2: EAT UP!

You're all psyched up, ready and raring to go. You've learned how to think, now it's time to address your eating habits. Food is fuel. Eating for any other reason causes weight gain. Plain and simple. This section is about getting back to the real purpose of food, getting real with the reasons you overeat and overindulge, and turning your diet around. You're about to kick-start your weight loss with a fuss-free meal plan that works!

Chapter 4: The Heads UP on Food for Fat Loss

At the end of day, diet is the most important factor in losing weight. There are plenty of people who frequent the gym regularly, play sports or walk everywhere, but still carry excess body fat. Weight loss aside, exercise remains essential for good health and quality of life, but unless you couple exercise with a disciplined approach to eating you won't get the weight-loss results you're after.

Eat less, move more

No matter what fancy foods you eat, what diet you go on, what fad you try, you can't escape the tried and tested and true rule of weight loss:

Calories in > Calories out = Weight gain

Calories in = Calories out = Weight maintenance

Calories in < Calories out = Weight loss

Consume more calories than you burn and you will gain weight; consume less calories than you burn and you will lose weight; consume the same amount of calories as you burn and you will most likely maintain your weight. In other words: if you eat up more than you burn up you will gain weight!

So how do we eat up less than we burn up?

'Calories in' come from what you eat and drink — pretty simple.

'Calories out' come from the energy you burn up through your basic daily movements and any exercise you do as well as the energy you burn by way of your resting metabolism.

Your resting metabolism, called your Basal Metabolic Rate (BMR), accounts for around 60–70 per cent of the calories you burn each day. So at rest, meaning outside of any physical movement you do, your body is busy burning calories — producing hormones, making new cells, regulating temperature, pumping your heart, and so on. Because your BMR accounts for such a sizeable chunk of the total calories you burn each day, you can see why it pays to have a speedy metabolism.

Rev up your metabolism

While our metabolic rate is already largely pre-determined, there are things you can do to help speed it up:

- Exercise at high intensities to create a prolonged after burn effect.

- Lift heavy weights to maintain lean muscle tissue (the more muscle the higher the metabolism).

- Eat small meals frequently to keep your metabolism stimulated.

By consuming less calories than you burn through your BMR, exercise and physical activity you will create what is called a calorie deficit — this is when you'll start to lose weight.

There are formulas to work out what calorie deficit an individual would have to make in order to lose weight based on the amount of energy that individual expends each day, but all you need to know is that if you reduce the amount of calories you eat (I've taken the guesswork out of it by advising on the best daily calorie quota to stick to for guaranteed weight loss in the Hard'n Up Meal Plan to follow), and move more, you will lose weight!

It's also important to remember that the body is a living, breathing organism geared for survival, it cares little about formulas and what science says it *should* lose in a week. Social, environmental, physical and mental states also have a profound effect on day-to-day weight loss.

You need to strip away those emotional, comforting, indulgent attachments to food and view it as a fuel that will allow you to get the most from your body and life.

'Fess up!

Food has become a drug that poisons lives. A large proportion of society has forgotten that food is a fuel source — and that's it! But people eat for so many other reasons.

- As a source of enjoyment.

- To distract themselves from boredom.

- As a procrastination tactic to avoid getting the hard things done.

- To ease emotional pain.

- As a way to celebrate occasions with friends, families ... anyone!

- Self-destruction stemming from a deeper issue (food addiction is no different to any other type of addiction, be it gambling, shopping, alcohol or drugs).

All of these reasons have clouded and obscured our true hunger signals — to eat only when we're physically (not emotionally or mentally) hungry and stop before we're overfull.

Eat what you need, not what you want.

It's time to 'fess up about the real reasons you eat!

Every time you feel like eating for any other reason other than genuine hunger, ask yourself the questions: 'Why am I eating now?' 'Am I bored, upset, stressed, depressed, unhappy, insecure?' The answers may not come straightaway. But if you pay attention to what's really eating you, instead of eating away the emotion, you will discover the real reasons behind your overeating. Then, you can choose to take non-food ways to deal with your thoughts and emotions. Like any skill, the more you practice doing this, the stronger your resolve and the better you get at it.

Emotional bookmarks

We all have emotional bookmarks, put in place at various chapters throughout our lives. A major one in emotional eaters stems back to childhood when food was given by our parents to soothe pain, as a reward or incentive for good behaviour, or to keep us quiet.

Scenario:

The child falls over and hurts themselves.

Parent's response:

'There, there, it will be all right, have a chocolate.'

Emotional bookmark:

Food makes me feel better; food soothes pain.

Scenario:

Going to the supermarket.

Parent's response:

'If you behave in the supermarket you can have a lollipop.'

Emotional bookmark:

Food is a reward; I've been good, I deserve a treat.

Scenario:

The child won't be quiet.

Parent's response:

'Sit in front of the TV, eat your snack and be quiet.'

Emotional bookmark:

Food is a distraction; eating food in front of the TV goes hand-in-hand.

The overall message is that food takes you to a better or happier or quieter place, helping you to avoid dealing with the real problem or issue as it arises. The belief is set up that food numbs pain.

Of course, this isn't about blaming your parents. Not all parents use food as a reward or form of distraction with their kids. We create our fair share of emotional bookmarks for ourselves as we grow up. For example, devouring a block of chocolate to get over a break-up creates the emotional bookmark that food helps deal with heartache and disappointment. Whatever your emotional bookmark or belief about food, wherever it came from, you need to break it and remove your emotional attachment to food.

If it helps you can seek the help of a weight-loss counsellor or the like to address these issues, but in my experience I've found that when people commit wholeheartedly to an eating and exercise program they innately have the mental tools to overcome their emotional eating issues on their own. All you need is some self-belief and to toughen up (with a cuddle thrown in along the way).

Breaking a lifetime of emotional bookmarks connected to food and poor eating habits is hard; I'm not discounting that. But one thing I know for sure is that nothing worth achieving ever comes easily — it takes the hard yards. So buckle up and commit to changing your diet, starting now.

The big guns of nutrition

Just like a car, your body needs fuel for energy in order to function. In your body this fuel is food. Just as there are different types of fuel for cars, there are different types of fuel for our bodies — carbohydrates, fats and protein. These are called the three macronutrients — or the big guns of nutrition.

To better understand the best foods for weight loss and peak performance, let's look at each of these big guns in a bit more detail.

For optimum performance you need optimum performance fuel. To help our bodies perform at their best we need fresh, healthy, nutritious food.

Slow and steady wins the diet race

When it comes to losing weight keeping your blood sugar levels nice and steady is imperative. The more foods we eat that cause a surge in blood sugar the more insulin the body releases to return blood sugar levels to normal. An excess of insulin promotes fat storage, which is not good for weight loss.

Also, when our blood sugar levels drop too low (remember Blue Team Philosophy number 4: what goes up must come down!) our bodies crave sugary, fatty foods to bring blood sugar levels back up, so you end up with a spike effect — again, not good for managing weight and cravings.

Too much sugar in the blood is also linked to a host of health problems, such as Type 2 diabetes, insulin resistance, obesity and heart disease.

Carbohydrates explained

Carbohydrates (most commonly known as 'carbs') are the body's preferred supply of energy — providing energy for our muscles to move, our brains to think, and our bodies to function. There are three categories of carbohydrates: simple carbohydrates, complex carbohydrates and dietary fibre. Or more simply: sugars, starches and fibre.

Simple carbohydrates (sugars)

Simple carbohydrates are absorbed into the bloodstream very quickly. Refined simple carbohydrates — think foods made from white sugar such as sweets, soft drink, pastries, cakes and cookies — give you a 'sugar rush' causing a fleeting energy boost before crashing and burning and dumping energy levels to lower than before. These types of sugars are linked to too much sugar and insulin in the body, diabetes and obesity, and should be avoided all together.

Naturally occurring simple sugars can be found in foods such as fruit and fruit juice, and vegetables. Although natural sugars can be good for you in terms of nutrients, too much sugar is not so good for you in terms of weight loss so all sugars, no matter what the source, need to be monitored.

Natural sugars found in tropical fruit can play havoc with blood sugar levels.

Complex carbohydrates (starches)

Unprocessed, natural sources of complex carbohydrates — think wholegrains, long grain brown rice, vegetables and legumes — take longer to be broken down and absorbed, making them the better choice for health and weight loss as they make you feel fuller for longer and don't cause a rapid rise in blood sugar.

Refined sources of complex carbohydrates on the other hand — think foods made from white flour such as pasta, pizza dough, cakes and white breads — are not good for weight loss and health as they are calorie dense and have had most of the goodness (nutrients) stripped and bleached away, and usually increase blood sugar and insulin.

Fibre for fat loss

We know fibre is a must for a happy digestive system and healthy bowel movements but it's also a must for weight loss. Fibre helps increase feelings of fullness, delays hunger, and keeps the all-important blood sugar levels stable by slowing the absorption of sugars after eating which helps manage appetite and control cravings.

Our daily fibre requirements are around 30 grams a day, but this can be hard to take in — for example, one slice of wholegrain bread only contains around 2 grams of fibre.

Some easy ways to meet your daily fibre intake

Sprinkle: Add high fibre sprinkles, such as All-bran or psyllium, to cereal, yoghurt and salad dressings.

Eat oats: Rolled oats are one of our fibre friends helping to keep us full and energetic over our morning so we don't feel tempted to reach for that biscuit with our mid-morning tea. Oats also help to lower cholesterol and maintain stable blood sugar levels.

Leave the skin on fruit: The skin has the most fibre.

Eat plenty of vegetables: Eat a wide variety of vegetables in all colours to maintain fibre intake.

Add raspberries to your oats, cereal or yoghurt: One cup of raspberries has around 8 grams of fibre, not to mention they are low in calories and high in antioxidants!

Love your legumes: Heart healthy beans and legumes score very high in the fibre stakes and do wonders for satisfying and sustaining appetite.

Choose bran-based cereals: You can even sprinkle some over low-fat yoghurt for a high fibre, high protein snack.

Eat your wholegrains: A wholegrain means all three parts of the original grain remain, so it hasn't had a lot of processing from its original form. A wholegrain can be a food on its own (for example, brown rice) or can be an ingredient in food (for example, soy and linseed bread contains wholegrain ingredients). Examples of less common wholegrains are quinoa and buckwheat — like rice, these are gluten free and make good wholegrain alternatives for those who can't stomach wheat.

If all else fails, use a fibre supplement: There are plenty on the market, including natural ones.

Note: When increasing fibre intake, be sure to drink plenty of water to avoid constipation.

'If you thir

or think y

you can,

u can't ...'

_____

Shannan Ponton

I recommend using the GI system of classifying carbohydrates. It is the best indicator of the response a carbohydrate will have on your system upon consumption. Glycaemic index (GI) is a measure of the effect that a food you eat has on your blood sugar. Foods are rated between 0–100, with foods rating closer to 100 releasing glucose relatively quickly compared to foods rated closer to 0.

- Foods with a GI of more than 70 are high GI, causing a rapid rise in blood sugar.

- Foods with a GI of 56–69 are moderate GI.

- Foods with a GI of less than 55 are low GI, causing the slowest rise in blood sugar.

We want the slowest surge in blood sugar and insulin for weight loss and health. The higher the GI, the greater the blood sugar and insulin spike. You can see why low GI foods are the way to go.

There are great pocket books and websites that tell you the GI of a wide range of foods.

Choosing carbohydrates for weight loss

- Eat low GI carbohydrates most (or all) of the time, moderate GI carbohydrates some of the time and avoid high GI carbs.

- Don't consume fruit by way of fruit juice or dried fruit, which are both high in calories and sugar.

- Stick to fruits that are lower in GI (remember even natural sources of sugar can be high GI and not helpful for weight loss). Low GI fruits include apples, grapefruit, lemons, oranges, plums, peaches, pears, blackberries, cherries, raspberries and strawberries.

- Stay away from tropical fruit. Generally, the sweeter the fruit the higher the sugar content tends to be.

- Eat a wide variety of vegetables but watch your intake of vegetables with a higher GI, particularly white potatoes — choose sweet potato (yam) instead which has a lower GI.

- When choosing breads and grains, think dark, heavy and grainy over white, light and fluffy. For example, multi-grain or soy and linseed bread over white bread; brown bulky rice over white fluffy rice.

- Choose long grain brown rice over white rice (even white rice that is low GI, such as Basmati). Brown rice is less processed so it retains more vitamins and minerals, and takes less volume (calories) to fill you up due to its higher fibre content, which will keep you feeling fuller for longer.

- Avoid pasta (white and wholemeal). Even though pasta has a moderate GI it is processed and therefore calorie dense.

- Always choose wholegrains with minimal processing (closest to its original form) such as oats instead of processed cereal.

- Keep your carbohydrate intake very low at night as you don't need very much energy to sleep!

Ideal Carbohydrate Intake for Weight Loss: Aim for a low carbohydrate intake in your overall meal plan (think 'low carbs', not 'no carbs').

Carbohydrates (mainly high GI carbs) can play havoc with your blood sugar, rapidly increasing insulin, which can single-handedly stop your body burning body fat! The best time to eat carbs is directly before activity or training, as you will burn them up.

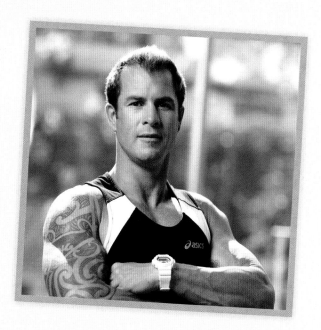

Fats explained

Fats are grouped into unsaturated (good fats) and saturated (bad fats). We need to include some fats in our diets in order to facilitate important functions, such as absorbing and using fat-soluble vitamins, and making hormones.

Monounsaturated, polyunsaturated and essential fatty acids (omega-6 and omega-3 fatty acids) are all unsaturated fats and when consumed in moderation can assist in good health and don't clog your arteries. Think seeds, olive oil and oily fish such as salmon.

Saturated fats such as full-fat dairy, palm oil and fatty meats, and trans fats (manufactured unsaturated fat that acts in the body in the same way as saturated fats) commonly found in pre-prepared commercial products such as margarine, fries, pies, pastries and doughnuts, are the bad guys in terms of health, cholesterol and your waistline. These types of fats are best removed from your diet all together.

Choosing fats for weight loss

- Buy lean meats and cold cuts with no visible fat through the meat.

- Always buy low- or no-fat dairy versions of cheese, milk and yoghurt.

- Avoid nuts, avocado, olives and oil-based dressings while losing weight. Although these are healthy fats, it's too tempting to eat more than you planned to and take in too many calories as a result.

- Oily fish such as salmon is okay as it provides a good dose of essential fatty acids. Because it tends to be higher in calories than other fish, aim for no more than two serves per week.

- When cooking use oil sprays instead, such as olive oil or canola spray, to save on calories.

Ideal Fat Intake for Weight Loss:
Aim for a low intake of all fats.

How many times have you said I'll just snack on a couple of nuts and before you know it you've ended up eating a handful! A small handful of nuts can have in excess of 180 calories! If you're on a 1200 calorie plan that's 15 per cent of your daily calorie intake gone — on just a few nuts!

Protein explained

Protein is used as a building block in the body, helping to build and repair muscle tissue, among many other functions.

Amino acids string together to make up protein. There are approximately 20 amino acids in the body, some the body manufactures on its own (non-essential amino acids), and some the body needs to get from food (essential amino acids because it's essential you eat them — pretty straightforwards).

Most animal foods provide all of the essential amino acids and are called complete proteins while plant foods often lack one or more of the essential amino acids making them incomplete proteins — this is important to know if you're vegetarian, as you need to combine different protein sources to make sure you're getting all the essential amino acids in your diet.

Including low-fat protein in your diet is essential for weight loss as it helps you to feel fuller for longer, stabilises blood sugar, which helps reduce cravings, and is not high in calories meaning you can fill up on protein without worrying about your weight.

Animal sources of protein include lean meats, poultry, eggs and low-fat dairy products. Non-animal protein sources include tofu, legumes and beans.

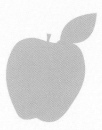

Choosing protein for weight loss

- Eat the egg white only (the yolk is high in fat, cholesterol and calories).

- Always choose low- or no-fat dairy products.

- Stick to low-fat cheeses/white cheeses, such as low-fat cottage cheese, as these are lower in cholesterol and fat.

- Eat plenty of chicken and turkey (no skin and preferably breast) as these are great low-fat sources of protein.

- When eating other meats, only buy lean cuts such as trim mince and lean steak. Avoid chops as it's too tempting to chew the fat instead of trimming it off and throwing away!

- Stick to low-fat cold meats such as ham, turkey and chicken (avoid salami or cold cuts with visible fat).

- Buy tinned tuna and salmon in springwater not oil.

- Eat plenty of white fish but keep oily fish such as salmon to no more than two serves a week due to the high fat and calorie content.

Ideal Protein Intake for Weight Loss:
Aim for a moderate–high protein intake in your overall meal plan.

Feed the man meat!

Many dieters baulk at the thought of meat for fear of the fatty sinew. But lean meats that have low amounts of fat, such as lean beef, chicken and turkey, are high in protein (helps you feel fuller for longer), are low in calories and are packed with important vitamins and minerals such as iron. So what are you waiting for? Fire up the barbie!

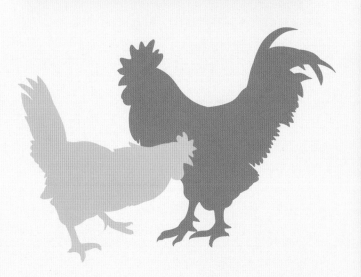

Diet secret revealed: not all calories are created equal

Fats are the most energy dense with 9 calories coming from 1 gram.

Protein and carbohydrates both provide 4 calories per 1 gram.

Alcohol yields 7 calories per 1 gram, but these are 'empty calories' meaning they have no nutritional value.

Fat, protein and carbohydrate are not all stored equally in the body. Fat is very easily converted to body fat and stored after consumption because it's already 'fat'. But if you have excess calories stored in the way of carbohydrates and protein, it's more difficult for the body to convert these calories and store them as body fat.

The massive chemical process of eating, digesting and converting food to be stored as body fat costs energy. When you have excess carbohydrates, you lose just under 50 per cent of the energy value of the food in the conversion process. When you have excess protein, you lose just over 50 per cent of the energy value in the conversion.

Use this to your advantage for weight loss — when you follow a high protein diet it is much harder for your body to store excess protein calories as fat.

That's why filling up on protein gives you a serious eating edge!

In regards to weight loss there is no difference between good fats and bad fats. As far as your butt and gut are concerned both have 9 calories per gram and if you consume too much fat (no matter what the source) it will end up going to your problem areas!

Chapter 5: Fuel UP — The Hard'n Up Meal Plan

The desire to eat is with you every minute that you're awake so there is constant pressure when trying to stick to a healthy eating regime. As in training, discipline is everything. You need a rock-solid, focused and committed attitude to resist the temptation of eating crap.

I have heard every excuse imaginable (none of which have ever swayed me) as to why people have succumbed to the desire to eat: 'My body tells me I need carbs'; 'There was nothing else at the football'; 'It was someone's birthday in the office'; 'It would've been rude not to have some cake'; 'I needed some good fat so I had half an avocado in my salad'; 'I was feeling tired so I had some jelly beans'; 'I thought I could have a Caesar salad as salad is healthy'; and on and on it goes.

All of the above (and all the others) are just excuses made to justify your poor eating choices when you're looking for an easy way out. If you really want to make a change you need to be honest about your eating habits (no more excuses) and face the fact that change will be hard at first, but the more you make better food choices the stronger you become and the easier it gets.

Stay strong!

One of the main reasons people can't lose weight is food, food and food! Our environments are such that there's temptation everywhere you turn — TV advertising, service station and grocery check-outs (also a major temptation to kids), social functions, morning and afternoon tea at work, dinner parties and the temptations we place around the home 'just in case guests come over'.

Set yourself up for success and rid your house of temptation. That's right, be brutal and throw out (or give away) EVERYTHING that should not be in your cupboard or fridge! That packet of biscuits, lollies or chips will never find its way to the starving people of the world — so get rid of it.

Don't be a victim of food. You must learn to say no and take control! Every time you do you take one step closer to achieving your goal and strengthening your commitment to a healthier, happier you!

About the meal plan — 8 diet philosophies

The Hard'n Up Meal Plan has been formulated from all my years in the fitness and weight-loss industry and guiding my teams and contestants on *The Biggest Loser*. I have found this diet and nutrition program to be the most effective and sustainable.

Longevity and sustainability are the two most important factors in dropping weight, staying healthy and keeping the weight off.

It's important to stress that the Hard'n Up Meal Plan isn't a diet because that implies you can go on and off it. You can't. You need to find a new way of eating for life.

As most of you know fad diets don't work long term. This is because most people return to their old eating habits once the diet is over. That's why the best and most effective way to maintain long-term weight loss is to modify your eating habits PERMANENTLY. This means finding low-fat, low-calorie, low GI foods that you like, fit in with your lifestyle and you can continue to eat indefinitely. The Hard'n Up Meal Plan introduces these foods and sets you on the right path for the future, giving you nutritious, healthy food to allow you to train and live.

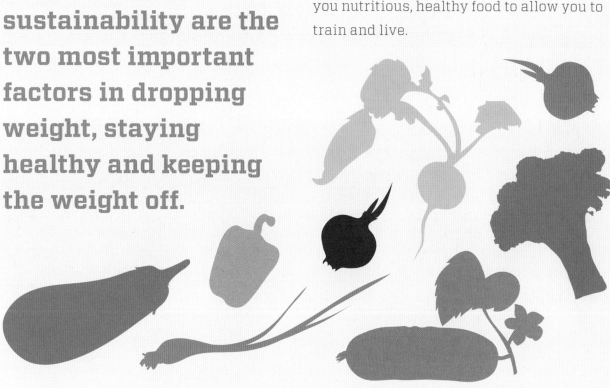

The meal plan is based on 8 diet philosophies:

1. **Eat more low-fat protein.**

2. **Choose less-processed, low-GI carbohydrates.**

3. **Use simple flavours.**

4. **Include a cheat meal.**

5. **Don't drink your calories.**

6. **You play, you pay!**

7. **Time your meals.**

8. **Count calories to begin.**

---

1. Eat more low-fat protein

Many successful, well-known diet plans are based on the protein principle because it gets results — just ask my contestants! Criticism for high-protein diets is aimed at the health risks associated with high intakes of protein, but these risks have more to do with high protein diets that include high intakes of saturated fats and not enough fruit and vegetables — neither of which are found in the Hard'n Up Meal Plan.

Filling up on low-fat, high-protein foods helps you lose weight in the following ways.

- Eating protein takes fewer calories to feel full than carbohydrates and fat.

- Protein helps you to feel fuller for longer.

- Protein has a positive effect on stable blood sugar.

- Eating protein actually burns calories to digest as it takes more energy to breakdown protein and store as fat than it does carbohydrate and fats.

- Protein is great for curbing cravings. Try snacking on boiled egg whites, tuna in springwater, low-fat cheese, a glass of skim milk or cold cuts of meat to stave off a craving — it works! (And not too many people have an emotional attachment to eating lean chicken!)

- Adequate protein is necessary for muscle growth, and for recovery and repair from exercise.

- Low-fat protein is low in calories and helps keep your overall calorie intake down.

Milk it, baby

We know that calcium is essential for strong bones and warding off osteoporosis, but you may not be aware of its perks for weight loss. Several large studies have found that a high calcium consumption of low-fat dairy products substantially aids weight loss. And yoghurt eaters lose more fat from their waist, making yoghurt the perfect go-to snack for weight loss!

2. Choose less-processed, low-GI carbohydrates

Carbohydrates give us energy to train, think, and live. But if you put too much carbohydrate in your tank it will end up being stored as fat. It's as basic as that.

That's why it's best to keep your carbohydrate consumption low, eating just enough to top up your energy stores to get you through training and your daily activities.

Overeating carbohydrates causes a surge of sugar and insulin, which causes a surge in appetite, preventing fat from being burnt up for energy, leading to fat storage.

Just as your car requires a specific fuel to function efficiently so does your body. The type of fuel you need to keep your body running while at the same time losing weight is low-GI carbohydrate with minimal processing — the majority of your carbohydrate intake must come from these types of carbs.

Ideally, consume your carbohydrates, especially fruit, before training to ensure you don't get left with excess carbohydrates that may get stored as fat if you don't burn them off.

Indulgent, decadent, calorie-laden food that leaves you craving more is the drug that ruins food addicts' lives.

3. Use simple flavours

If you're looking for loads of tasty meals that will wow your tastebuds (but throw your weight loss into a tail spin), you're not going to find them in this meal plan. The meals are simple, fuss-free and keep rich flavours to a minimum. But don't run away just yet … there's a reason for this.

If you eat a plain-tasting meal that doesn't make your tastebuds dance and sing and jump for joy, do you want to overeat or go back for seconds or thirds? Not likely. Now think about your favourite indulgent meal that makes you think for that moment that heaven has been dished up on a plate. How much more likely are you to overindulge and go back for seconds and thirds?

If something tastes that good it's hard to stop at just a small serving. No one's suggesting you eat food that tastes bad — just not so irresistible that you can't stop yourself from overindulging on the types of food that don't support your health and weight-loss goals!

Your body needs food to function so feed it basic food, enough to top up your energy stores and then move on until your next top-up meal or snack. The goal is to view food as a source of fuel rather than a source of pleasure.

To do this you need to retrain your tastebuds. If you keep feeding your tastebuds sugar, salt and all sorts of fancy flavours, you're conditioning those little tastebuds to want more. Just as you need to train your muscles to get used to activity and exercise (a different way of living), you have to train your tastebuds to get used to simple, healthy food (a different way of eating).

By keeping your flavours simple for a good amount of time you will retrain your tastebuds to appreciate good, healthy food. In time, you won't have to use willpower to choose healthy meals: your tastebuds will naturally take you there because that's what they will crave and want.

When I first recommend that people avoid rich flavours and eat simple meals, the suggestion is usually met with serious resistance. 'That's boring', is the usual reaction. In fact, many a person has told me that I'm boring because of the way I eat. To this my response is along the lines of: 'If food is what defines me, then shoot me! What makes me exciting is the person I am, not the food I do or do not eat. I get excitement from the adventurous life I lead.'

The truth is when you show enough strength of character to resist foods that are not good for your health or weight loss you feel empowered and good, not boring. Eating healthily allows you to have a much happier, enriched life. This means much, much, MUCH more than any indulgent meal! As the saying goes, 'Nothing tastes as good as fit and healthy'.

Whether you're an athlete, weekend warrior or morbidly obese, to achieve your goals, taste and the momentary satiety you enjoy from eating must take a back seat to optimum nutrition. There are plenty of other places to take enjoyment from other than food, such as spending quality time with friends and family, hobbies, vacations, adventure sports, achieving your goals and so on.

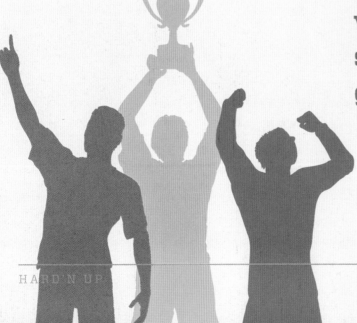

Shannan's typical daily diet

Breakfast

- ⅓ cup oats
- Sportsedge ('Natures way') protein whey powder
- Low sugar, low-fat yoghurt
- Mixed berries

Mid-morning snack

- One piece of non-tropical fruit, such as an apple or orange

Lunch

- 200g chicken with steamed vegies (microwave bag)
- ½ cup long grain brown rice

Afternoon snack

- ⅓ cup Goodness Superfoods P1 protein cereal
- Protein powder
- 1 tub diet/light yoghurt

Dinner

- Lean meat and vegies such as chicken and vegie stir-fry, barbecued chicken breast or white fish such as barramundi or basa or lean meat with a big plate of salad or a mountain of vegies.

My indulgences

- Mum's home-cooked Chinese once a week (it's been a family tradition for 20 years!)
- Mum's desserts
- Chicken burgers (I get two grilled chicken breasts, pull the guts out of the roll, ask for extra salad, fresh chilli and no mayo. Who said healthy eating was boring?)

'Being fit an
weight cou
life; it's that

a healthy
save your
serious!'

———————————

Shannan Ponton

4. Include a cheat meal

If the thought of eating only plain and simple food is hard to swallow, there's a little light at the end of the week's diet tunnel. You get to eat a cheat meal where you can eat whatever you like. The 'cheat meal' tactic is helpful for maintaining long-term consistent weight loss because it psychologically gives you something to look forwards to in the short term and you don't feel resentful about giving up everything.

But it's only one meal per week! Not two or three. Just one. A cheat meal can be anything you like that strays from the set menu plan or Approved List of Foods (see Chapter 6). One meal means one serving, for example: one hamburger, one slice of cheesecake, one blueberry muffin, one serving of hot chips, one bowl of pasta, one ice-cream cone, one chocolate bar — you get the gist. You'll be able to gauge how much you can 'get way with' without impacting on your weight loss quite quickly. But the key thing to remember is that the cheat meal isn't a permission slip to hoe down an all-you-can-eat buffet or to overindulge in a second or third helping.

One of the most common diet misconceptions is that if you've been really 'good' all week you can let loose on the weekend. This is an absolute no-no. If you do this, you'll almost always put back on any weight that you've lost during the week.

Each week you set yourself a treat. This might be popcorn at the movies, garlic bread at the Italian restaurant with friends, a muffin with your skim latte on Monday morning, dessert at Friday night's dinner party, Mum's baked dinner with gravy and so on.

You'll look forward to your cheat meal and savour every mouthful like you've probably never done before. (Think about it. How many times have you scoffed down a big bag of potato chips while watching TV because your attention was focused on the TV and not on what you were eating?) With a cheat meal, because you know you don't get another one for a whole week, you really will make it last as long as possible.

Once you're committed to your eating and exercise plan you may feel guilty when you have your cheat meal, but the feeling will pass in a few days. Then you'll spend the next few days looking forward to the next cheat meal before getting satisfaction again.

As you get further along in your weight loss you may even find that your choice of cheat meal becomes healthier and healthier. You may see a full-fat yoghurt or cappuccino with full-cream milk as your cheat meal (*Yeah right,* I hear you thinking, but don't underestimate just how empowered and good you're going to feel once you've cleaned up your diet and are losing weight). Once you retrain your tastebuds to appreciate much simpler foods with less richness, you'll find many foods are much too rich to eat when you previously didn't. As a result, you'll naturally go for less rich versions without thinking about it, such as oven-baked wedges over deep-fried chips.

5. Don't drink your calories

Keeping hydrated is essential for good health, maximising exercise performance and maintaining metabolism. But you don't need to consume calories to hydrate.

Many people come unstuck by drinking their calories instead of eating them: using full-fat milk in tea and coffee, adding cream and syrups to takeaway coffee, drinking soft drink, consuming too much juice or fruit smoothies, choosing high-calorie alcoholic drinks like pre-mixed drinks, creamy cocktails and standard beers.

People are either unaware of just how much sugar and calories are in soft drinks, cordials and alcohol, or can be lulled into a false sense of security when drinking fresh juice or fruit smoothies because they're 'healthy' — they may have healthy ingredients but they can contain just as much sugar and calories as soft drink.

When it comes to hydrating, water is your best source.

6. You play, you pay!

Remember everything comes at a cost. And in weight-loss terms the currency is calories. Learn the debt you need to pay back when you overindulge. If you've had a night out and eaten a couple slices of pizza washed down with a couple beers or wines, a one-hour walk isn't going to come even close to repaying this debt; you'd more likely need to power walk for three to four hours! Once you work out how much extra exercise you have to do to pay for your binges you'll soon realise it's much easier not to overindulge in the first place.

7. Time your meals

Planning set meal times is an effective way to prevent overeating and keep blood sugar levels stable. The average person is up for 16 hours a day, if you divide 16 by five (meals), you get 3.2 making the ideal time span between meals, every three hours. If you plan set meal times every 3 hours from the time you get up and have breakfast, you not only ensure you don't miss a meal and have your blood sugar levels drop — leaving you starving and more likely to your crave the wrong foods — you'll be less likely to gorge because you know you have another meal coming in 3 hours' time. Timing meals will truly help you take control of your cravings. Stick to the clock, it'll never let you down!

8. Count calories to begin

In an ideal world we would instinctively know what to eat to best serve our health, eat only when we're hungry and stop before we're overfull. But living in a society with a surplus of poor food choices means many people have lost sight of these natural instincts. That's why we need to count and calculate our calories; because we have a tendency to underestimate how much food we eat (not to mention overestimate how much exercise we do!). You'll only need to do this at first because your natural instincts will eventually kick in and you'll be able to choose wisely without referring to a calorie counter or calculator.

Always check the calorie amounts of new foods and ingredients you introduce. Calorie amounts for basic foods are allocated in the menu plan. For other foods/ingredients refer to a calorie counting book or calorie counter online.

Eating and exercise

A common question is 'Does exercising in the morning before breakfast burn more fat?' The answer is yes and no. It's true that doing a workout before breakfast can help tap into your fat stores for energy better than doing a workout after breakfast as your glucose stores are low (your body's first source of energy when working out) from not eating for 8 or more hours overnight, forcing the body to go to the next in line for energy supply: fat stores. But here's the catch: If you haven't eaten anything for 4 to 5 hours before training low blood sugar can make you feel dizzy or faint, making it hard to exercise at high intensities, so although you might be burning more fat you won't be burning as many overall calories because you're not able to train at a high intensity, and the more calories you burn the more fat you lose.

In a nutshell: exercise before breakfast is fine for lighter intensity training, providing you don't feel dizzy or faint, but if you want to do a hard workout or a heavy weights session it's best to have a light snack within an hour of training so your exercise performance won't be affected from not having enough energy stores to keep up with the demands of the workout.

A basic guide on eating before exercise

- Exercise before breakfast on an empty stomach (providing you don't get dizzy) when doing low-intensity training.

- Eat carbohydrates within an hour before doing high-intensity training.

A basic guide on eating after exercise

- You can get away with not eating for 1 to 2 hours after doing a low-intensity session such as yoga, Pilates or a light walk to increase the fat and calories burned.

- Don't eat for an hour after doing moderate to high intensity training to help your body burn the calories and fat from the workout before replacing them, unless you're training specifically for athletic performance where it's important to replace your glycogen stores within 30 minutes to aid recovery so you can back up for the next training session and perform at the optimum level.

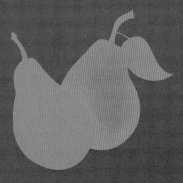

Diet foods

Choosing reduced fat, sugar, salt and calorie versions of healthy foods assists weight loss. Some examples of these include no-fat yoghurt, sugar-free cereal, diet sauces and dressings, low-carb beer, low-cal wine and so on. When choosing these types of products be sure to read the ingredients list and not just the claims — 'low fat', 'no sugar', 'half the calories', etc — splashed across the label to make sure the food is low in sugar, fat and calories. For example, some products might be low in fat but not sugar and calories (most lollies are 99 per cent fat free but are very high in sugar and low-sugar chocolate might still be 30 per cent fat). Also check to see if the food contains artificial sweeteners if you prefer to avoid these. While there is much debate about the safety and effectiveness of artificial sweeteners found in some diet foods, I do believe products such as diet soft drink, diet cordial and diet desserts are beneficial for those times when you just can't beat a craving for something sweet.

Meal plan guidelines

The menu plans have been formulated to get results. Although there's a big selection of diverse and varied healthy foods and flavours available in the market, the foods selected for the plans have been chosen because they are simple and accessible, and, most importantly, are tried and tested to be most conducive to your weight loss. The foods and menu plans are the same ones given to my *Biggest Loser* contestants.

If you want to include a food that's not on the menu plan the answer is most likely 'no', however, given that I'm not a food connoisseur and can't predict everyone's food preferences according to their culture or health choices/requirements (vegetarian, vegan, gluten-free, dairy-free, etc), you may need to add or replace some foods. If this is the case, you must do your research (use the internet, a calorie-counting book or seek dietary advice from a professional) to make sure it fits the following criteria.

- Matches or is less than the calorie amount of the approved food/meal you're replacing.

- Is swapped for the same category of food, that is, you can only replace a carbohydrate with a carbohydrate, a protein with a protein.

- Are always low GI, low sodium (salt), low fat and low sugar.

- If adding to the unlimited list of approved salad and vegetables it must be less than 10 grams carbohydrate per 100 grams, trace only fat and protein, approximately 25 to 40 calories per 100 grams, and low GI.

Keep in mind that this menu plan works and the more you deviate from it, the greater the risk of not getting your desired results.

Daily calorie quota

My contestants on *The Biggest Loser* have always followed a low-calorie menu plan that meets most of the Recommended Dietary Intake (RDI) requirements recommended by dieticians. Low-calorie diet plans are sometimes criticised but providing you meet your nutritional requirements, a low-calorie diet is acceptable and very effective. It encourages rapid weight loss, which increases the motivation brought on by the weight-loss results, which strengthens the determination to stick to the plan, which encourages the desire for further results, further motivation, further determination, and so on and so on.

Low-calorie diets are not only effective for weight loss, they have also been found to offer several health benefits and increase life expectancy.

The menu plans work off the following calorie limits.

Women: 1000–1200 calories per day for weight loss **(never going lower than 1000 calories)**; 1200–1400 calories per day for maintenance.

Drinks guide

Here are some guidelines for making smart beverage choices for weight loss and including drinks in the Hard'n Up Meal Plan.

Water: Drink around eight glasses a day and top up before, during and after a training session. When you exercise regularly it's imperative to stay well hydrated, especially in hot weather. As a rule for medium- to high-intensity training you need 150–200ml every 20 minutes especially if exercising in a hot environment or outdoors.

Juice

Remember, although fruit is good for you it's a form of sugar (calories) and to make juice you need to condense many pieces of fruit just to get one glass, which translates to a lot of sugar (calories). For example, one glass of orange juice can contain double the amount of calories of one small orange (your hunger would be much more satisfied eating an orange than gulping a glass of orange juice. Also, juice doesn't have the fibre content of fruit, and fibre is necessary to slow down the absorption of the sugar from the fruit. It's best to keep away from juice when losing weight.

Smoothies

If you drink a smoothie you need to count it as a meal or snack (not as an additional beverage) and work the calories into your daily quota accordingly.

Soft drinks and cordial

Go for diet soft drink or diet cordial. If you don't want to consume diet products with artificial sweeteners steer clear of soft drink and cordial completely. Try still or sparkling mineral water with a squeeze of fresh lemon, lime or orange.

Coffee and tea

If you drink coffee and tea you need to make sure you're not drinking added calories along with it: use no-fat milk, no sugar (or sugar replacers), and don't add toppings and syrups on offer from some takeaway coffee shops. Herbal teas without milk and sugar are fine.

Alcohol

Excess alcohol will impair your weight loss as it slows your metabolism, plays havoc with blood sugar, and increases the temptation to overeat or indulge in fatty foods — that pie and beer at the footy, that doner kebab on the way home, that extra garlic bread and pizza to soak up the wine, that bag of nuts or crisps you didn't even notice eating at the bar, that greasy breakfast to shake a hangover.

I love a beer as much as the next bloke, but if you're going to enjoy a drink or two you need to work it in to your calorie quota for the day/meal plan your consumption wisely and stay in control. If you're drinking with a meal or when you are out socialising, make sure you calculate the calories as part of the total meal.

If you do drink, always go for the low-calorie options such as low-carb beer, spirits with soda water and fresh lime or lemon (not lime/lemon cordial or syrup), spirits with diet soft drink or a small glass of wine (many wine glasses hold a lot more than the standard serve). Do not drink cocktails, creamy drinks, pre-mixed spirits in cans and bottles or spirits with non-diet soft drink — these are all very high in sugar and calories.

The recommended guidelines in Australia are no more than two standard drinks per day for women, and four for men, and at least two alcohol-free days each week. A standard drink contains 10 grams of pure alcohol. Read the bottle's label to find out the number of standard drinks it contains.

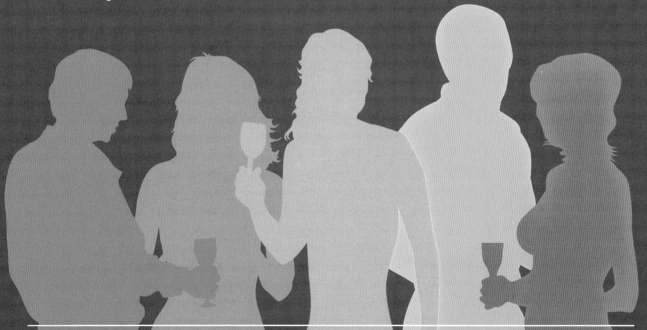

Men: 1200–1400 per day for weight loss **(never going lower than 1200 calories)**; 1400–1800 calories per day for maintenance.

Start on the lowest end of the calorie quota (1000–1200 for women, 1200–1400 for men) until you reach your desired weight loss. Then, gradually add calories without exceeding the upper end of the quota (1400 calories for women, 1800 calories for men) to the amount where you can maintain your weight. A simple rule for finding your maintenance quota is to gradually increase your calories; if you put on weight, even a kilo, you need to reduce your calories until your weight stays the same — this is your maintenance level.

Many diet plans recommend cutting your calories gradually, starting on a higher calorie-controlled plan before working your way down to a lower calorie plan, but by jumping straight to a lower calorie diet you will kick-start your weight loss, getting rapid results, which will give you incentive to keep going.

Also, when you factor in the extra calories from your weekly cheat meal, not to mention the inevitable slip-ups you'll have along the way (we're only human), your calorie intake will most likely end up within a higher range and not always fall in the lowest range.

The calorie amount of each food/meal is provided in the menu plan so it's up to you to work through and add up the calories of your choices to equate to your daily calorie quota. Remember, this is just to begin with until you've got your eating habits down pat and can instinctively know what to choose.

Creating your own plan within the guidelines is important because if a diet plan has set meals you may not always feel like what's on the menu that day or have those ingredients in your cupboard. The biggest part of this process is educating yourself — on the best foods to eat for weight loss and having a slim body for life; on the calorie amounts of the foods you eat; on how to put together a day of eating that best serves your health and weight; and where to make adjustments when you slip up, eat more than you planned to or take in extra unplanned calories when you are eating out.

If you do slip up by eating too big a portion size or something that's not on the allowed list, you need to adjust your calories for the rest of the day accordingly or work it off with extra exercise (remember diet philosophy number 6: you play, you pay!) to compensate and stay within the set daily calorie quota. It's important to note that this doesn't apply to your weekly cheat meal — it's a gloves off, eat-what-you-like, savour-every-mouthful, cheat meal (remember, one meal, not many cheat meals and definitely not an entire cheat day!) — then, get **straight back** to the menu plan.

Eating out and in

Cooking at home is ideal because you can control the amount of fat and calories that go into your meal and you always know exactly what you're eating. But we all have days where we're exhausted and don't feel up to preparing a home-cooked meal or packing our lunch, and we certainly can't avoid social get-togethers as they're a part of everyday life.

While most of your meals should be prepared by yourself or someone you trust, some of your meals can come from restaurants and takeaway places, providing you know how to make the right choices. Here are some tips to help you navigate your way through cafés, restaurants and takeaway menus without sabotaging your diet.

Eating out

The two main reasons people come unstuck when eating out is being faced with too much temptation or eating more calories than you planned to because you underestimate the amounts of fat and sugars contained within the meal.

When eating at a restaurant or café, you have a right as a customer to ask for the meals to be prepared how you want. You can ask for meals to be cooked without butter, for dressing on the side, to hold the mashed potato, and so on.

If a meal comes with something you're not supposed to be eating such as fries, ask for no fries because if they end up in the plate in front of you and you don't have the strength to say no, they will end up in your tummy!

Be smart enough and strong enough to order what you need.

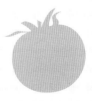

The same goes for parties, birthdays, functions and dinner parties. It's okay to ask the host to hold off on the fatty side dishes and sauces. And as far as being afraid to offend anyone by saying no, the person you're offending most is yourself by not standing up for your health.

Tips for eating out without coming unstuck

- Skip the bread if it's on the table when you sit down, or ask for some green salad instead.

- Ask for your meal to be cooked without butter or too much oil.

- Always get dressings and sauces on the side so you can control how much you take in (or eat your meal without dressings and sauces).

- Fill up on vegies and salad (make sure the vegies aren't cooked in butter — you can ask for them to be steamed or cooked with a little olive oil instead).

- Most restaurants have grilled chicken or fish on the menu and these are great choices.

- Go for tomato-based sauces and avoid the creamy sauces.

- Stick to the same meal times. If you eat dinner at 6 p.m. every day and dinner is booked at 8 p.m. you may end up overeating because you're too hungry.

- Do not eat three courses; one is best or you could have two entrée-sized meals.

- If you're drinking wine or beer with your meal, factor this into the overall calorie amount of the meal.

- Stick to protein (fish, chicken, pork, lamb, steak) plus salad and it will be hard to go wrong. Be sure to trim any excess fat that comes with the meat.

- Choose the protein that is grilled or baked, not fried or covered in batter.

- Stay away from the white stuff such as mashed potato, bread, pasta, noodles, rice or pizza bases as it's just too tempting to overeat these foods and consume too many calories.

- At parties never eat fried finger food and go for the healthiest option, for example: satay chicken or lean beef skewers (remove excess sauce), celery and carrot sticks instead of chips and dip, or low-fat cold cut meats — and always drink low-calorie drinks. If there's nothing healthy available say no and go without, it won't kill you, in fact, it will build discipline.

You are the customer and you have the right to order your preference. If you're met with resistance, try a new restaurant.

Eating in

Many fast-food chains are responding to consumer need for fast, fresh and healthy takeaway by adding and/or improving menu options. When ordering takeaway, do your homework first and get to know the ingredients and calories of your takeaway choices. Find places you know will serve you what you want.

Here are some good takeaway choices

- Healthy choice/low fat options are offered at many fast-food chains, do your research.

- Chicken kebab without the bread (a kebab plate).

- Barbecued chicken and salad (remove the skin and stick to the breast meat which is the leanest part).

- Grilled fish (check it's not coated in butter before grilling) with salad (definitely no chips).

- Asian takeaway: go for a stir-fry with the least amount of sauce, such as soy and ginger, skip the rice and noodles to compensate for the extra calories in the sauces and cooking methods.

- Thai takeaway: go for chicken satay sticks but ask for no sauce or sauce on the side (use very sparingly or not at all as satay sauce is high in fat and calories) or a Thai beef salad.

- Café breakfast: hard-boiled eggs (remove the yolk before eating) with grainy toast (no butter) or an egg white omelette with vegies like tomato and mushroom. It might take a bit of convincing to get the omelette made with just egg whites but all cafés should do this for you (if not, try a different café).

- Sandwiches: always ask for grainy bread and no butter, and stuff it with tuna or chicken and loads of salad. Scrape the fluffy centre out of bread rolls as this dramatically reduces calories and excess carbs and creates extra room for the good stuff — more protein and salad.

When eating rolls and healthy burgers, scrape the guts (dough) out of the roll to make a 'gutless roll' and save on calories!

Eating checklist

Here's a summarised checklist of all the dietary things you have to do to make sure you're on the right track (come back to this list to check that you're still on track throughout your weight-loss journey).

- I'm eating little to no processed foods.

- I go for low-GI carbs all of the time, moderate-GI carbs some of the time and avoid high-GI carbs altogether.

- I eat at least five servings of vegetables each day.

- I eat at least one, but no more than two, serves of fruit a day.

- I only eat my fruit in the morning or half an hour before training (a sprinkle of low-calorie berries at night is okay).

- I watch my intake of natural sugars that are a higher GI such as mangos, bananas, pineapple, dried fruit and fruit juice.

- I watch my intake of vegetables with a higher GI such as white potato, pumpkin, and corn.

- I always eat wholegrain breads, such as multi-grain and soy and linseed, instead of white bread.

- I avoid white sugars and starches such as two-minute noodles, crisps, pasta, white rice, rice crackers, potatoes, white flour, products made with white sugar (such as lollies and soft drink) and products made with white flour (such as pastries and biscuits).

- I eat long-grain brown rice instead of white rice.

- I eat oats, bran or protein enriched cereal instead of sugary cereals.

- I buy lean meat and always trim visible fat off my meat.

- I remove the skin from my chicken and stick to the breast meat, which is the leanest part.

- All of my dairy or soy products are low or no fat.

- I only eat the egg white, not the yolk.

- My main protein sources are lean chicken, turkey, egg whites and white fish.

- I snack mainly on low-fat cold meats, tuna in springwater, vegies such as beans, carrots and cucumber with low-fat cottage cheese, low-fat or diet yoghurt with some All-bran or oats stirred through (optional), or salad.

- I keep my carbohydrate intake very low at night.

- The bulk of my evening meal is always protein and vegies or salad.

- I use minimal oils in my cooking.

- I choose diet cordials, diet ice-cream, reduced sugar and fat products when I'm craving sugars, fats and/or carbs.

- I always choose low or no fat alternatives of foods, such as low-fat cheeses, skim milk, meats, and dressings.

I avoid nuts, avocado, olives, butter, cream and margarine because a fat is a fat in weight-loss terms.

I dress salad with vinegar instead of oil or low calorie/fat dressings.

I count calories to make sure I'm sticking to my daily calorie quota.

I make up for extra calories I've consumed with extra exercise.

I take the time to educate myself on the calorie amount of new foods I introduce or want to try and work it in to my overall daily calorie quota.

If you can tick off most of these you're doing well and are most likely losing weight. If you can tick off all of these you're doing an amazing job and are most certainly losing weight.

Supplements on the side

These are the basics I believe are essential for overall good health. Everyone has different dietary and supplementation needs and always seek professional advice before commencing supplementation. Individuals may benefit from a more comprehensive range of supplements, taking into account personal conditions and deficiencies.

- Multi-vitamin and mineral
- Fish oil
- Magnesium and zinc (particularly for males)
- Joint restore triple action for anyone experiencing inflamed, aching joints

Here are the supplements that I use daily, taken with breakfast and dinner (one tablet each twice a day, except for two tablets of garlic plus C and horseradish and double strength odourless fish oil, twice a day:

- Multivitamin (I use SuperNutrient mens Multi). Let's be honest, we all have days that are less than perfect and our nutrition suffers. Look for a multivitamin with a good make up of vitamins, minerals, and antioxidants (as a bonus).

- Joint Restore Triple Action. (A great mix of glucosamine+chondroitin+ Msm.) This product is for joint health, and after 30 years of training I need it.

- Garlic plus C and Horseradish. To boost immune function and prevent colds, hayfever and respiratory complaints.

- Active magnesium (Bioglan). To relieve muscular aches and cramps and assist sleeping.

- Chelated zinc (220mg). Assists in immune function, healthy skin and male reproduction.

- Max Q10+L-Carnitine. Recommended for heart health, boosting energy and assists in fat utilisation.

- Fish oil (2000mg). Beneficial for heart health, joints, brain function, eyes and general good health.

Chapter 6:
Plate UP —
Menu Plans

The Hard'n Up Meal Plan is designed to remove emotional bookmarks from food and allow you to view food as a fuel — done mechanically (timed by the hour) it will become something you just do — it will give you the power to overcome your food demons and the tools to keep them silenced.

Because the plan is about choosing a new way of eating that you will stick to for life, you have the flexibility to mix and match your own meals. You can prepare any meals you like using the Approved List of Foods below, providing you stick within the calorie quota per day.

Approved list of foods

You'll notice that many foods that are good for you, such as nuts, avocado, olives and some fruit and vegetables, don't appear on the list for the simple fact that they're not so good for you when trying to lose weight, due to their high calorie, fat and/or sugar content.

Remember, to lose weight our overall objective is to keep our sugar, fat and calorie count low.

You may notice that some of the foods fall into more than one category. For example, vegetables are a type of carbohydrate but not the same type of carbohydrates you have to worry about when it comes to weight loss such as white starches and sugars. You'll also see legumes/ beans under the carbohydrate category even though they're also a good source of protein (especially for vegetarians). Again, because we're trying to keep calories low, legumes/ beans must be kept to no more than one serve a day and considered in carbohydrate terms. There are many other foods that are both a carbohydrate and protein and also contain small amounts of fat such as low-fat dairy, but are grouped under the category that makes most sense when combining meals for weight loss.

You can also use the Approved List of Foods as a shopping list. Make a copy of the list and circle or highlight the foods you need to pick up for the week or write them out as a separate shopping list.

Approved salads

Tomato, capsicum, lettuce (all types), rocket, baby spinach, celery, mushroom, cucumber, carrot, onions (all types), radish, sprouts/bean sprouts, fennel.

Approved salad dressings

- Fat-free salad dressings (use sparingly).

- Balsamic vinegar, to taste.

- Lemon juice, to taste.

Approved salad suggestions

- Mixed leaf salad: mix of any green leaves plus a squeeze of lemon juice plus cracked black pepper.

- Tomato salad: chopped tomatoes plus diced Spanish onion plus torn fresh basil plus a splash of balsamic vinegar.

- Mixed salad: any type of lettuce plus mixed vegetables plus no-fat/low-calorie dressing.

- Baby spinach salad: baby spinach leaves plus sliced red onion plus roasted capsicum and mushroom (sliced and then grilled) plus a splash of balsamic vinegar plus cracked black pepper.

Note: Unlimited approved salad vegetables allowed as they all have less than 10 grams carbohydrate per 100 grams, trace only fat and protein, approximately 25–40 calories per 100 grams.

Approved vegetables

Broccoli, carrot, mushrooms, beans, cabbage, cauliflower, peas, snow peas, beans, asparagus, zucchini, brussels sprouts, bok choi, broccolini, choi sum, squash, spinach, leek.

Approved methods for cooking vegetables

- Raw.

- Steam — steamer or microwave.

- Boil.

- Stir-fry in non-stick frypan.

- Grill.

- Bake — lightly coat with oil spray if needed.

Approved vegetable suggestions

- Steamed vegetables plus a squeeze of lemon plus cracked black pepper or chilli.

- Stir-fried Asian greens plus garlic plus a splash of low-salt soy sauce.

- Baked vegetables coated in spray oil and chopped fresh parsley.

- Capsicum, mushroom, asparagus and/or zucchini, cut into strips and grilled.

- Vegetables of choice simmered in 100 per cent natural, salt-reduced tomato pasta sauce or tinned tomatoes plus a sprinkle of low-fat cottage cheese on top (as per protein allowance).

- Boiled cauliflower mashed with low-fat cottage cheese (as per protein allowance) plus cracked black pepper.

- Sliced cabbage, garlic and leek fried in a non-stick frypan plus cracked black pepper or a sprinkle of paprika.

- Vegetable soup: dry fry garlic and chopped onion (use a spray of oil if needed) in non-stick frypan, add low-salt vegetable stock, vegetables and a bay leaf (optional), bring to the boil, reduce to simmer and cook until vegetables are soft.

Note: Unlimited approved vegetables allowed as all have less than 10 grams carbohydrate per 100 gram, trace only fat and protein, approximately 25–40 calories per 100 grams.

Approved protein

- Eggs (egg whites only).

- Tins of tuna (in springwater or brine or low-fat, flavoured tuna).

- Tins of salmon (in springwater or brine).

- White fish and fresh tuna.

- Salmon, fresh (no more than 2 serves a week).

- Chicken (preferably breast), skinless.

- Turkey (preferably breast), skinless.

- Lean pork loin chops.

- Lean steak.

- Leg of lamb.

- Cold cuts of low-fat meat (low-fat ham, turkey, chicken, roast beef).

- Low-fat dairy: diet yoghurt, low-fat cheese, low-fat cottage cheese, low- or no-fat milk, etc.

- Low-fat calcium-fortified soy (low-fat or fat-free soy milk, low-fat soy yoghurt).

- Tofu.

Approved cooking methods

- Barbecue — use a spray of oil if needed.

- Grill.

- Dry fry in a non-stick frypan.

- Bake/Roast — use a spray of oil if needed.

- Steam.

Note: See menu plan for daily allowance.

Approved desserts

- Nestlé diet dessert.

- Diet/low-fat yoghurt.

- Nestlé Peter's no added sugar ice-cream.

- Cottee's diet topping.

- Sprinkle of berries.

Note: This is an optional inclusion for those who have a sweet tooth and still feel they need that 'full stop' after dinner.

Approved fruits

- Apple.

- Orange.

- Peach.

- Pear.

- Plum.

- Berries — strawberries, blackberries, blueberries, raspberries.

- Grapefruit.

Note: All fruits are low GI. Eat at least one serve a day, but no more than two serves a day.

Approved carbohydrates

- All-bran.

- Oats.

- 'Goodness Superfoods' P1 (Protein 1st) or D1 (Digestive 1st) cereal (a low-GI wholegrain cereal range found at most supermarkets).

- Sweet potato (yam).

- Multi-grain bread.

- Seed and grain bread, such as Bürgen soy and linseed.

- Long-grain brown rice.

- Legumes/beans: soy beans, lentils, chickpeas, butter beans, lima beans, broad beans, kidney beans.

Note: One serve at breakfast plus one serve at lunchtime (additional small spoonfuls of All-bran added to yoghurt allowed for morning and afternoon snack).

Approved flavourings

- Herbs.

- Chilli.

- Garlic.

- Pepper.

- Lemon juice.

- Low-sodium soy sauce.

- Diet/low-fat/low-calorie dressings and condiments.

Note: Use any to flavour foods instead of using salt and/or oil. Double check any diet or low-fat/low-calorie dressings to make sure they are actually low in both calories and fat. Factor calories from added flavourings into the calorie count for the meal (not necessary for herbs, chilli, garlic, and pepper as these are low in calories and used only in small amounts).

Approved fats

- Canola oil spray.

- Olive oil spray.

Note: You get enough incidental fat per day through foods like seeds (in soy and linseed bread), tuna and salmon, low-fat dairy and so on. Add a spray of oil when cooking if and where needed.

Converting favourite recipes

- Take the oils out of the recipe and replace with spray oil if necessary.

- Remove unnecessary added fats such as nuts, avocado, olives, cream and butter.

- Replace sauces and dressings with diet and reduced-salt/low-sodium versions.

- Remove sugars and replace with low-calorie sweeteners.

- Omit white starchy carbohydrates such as white rice, pasta, potatoes, flour and bread.

- Use lean protein sources.

Approved snacks

- Raw vegetable sticks or pieces (from approved vegetables) dipped in low-fat cottage cheese.

- Approved salads.

- Low-fat tuna.

- Low-fat cold cuts of meat served on its own or rolled up with grated vegetables and low-fat cottage cheese.

- Diet or low-fat yoghurt.

- Diet or low-fat yoghurt with All-bran.

- Low-GI fruit.^

Note: Two snacks per day.

^At least one serve, no more than two serves, a day due to sugar content of fruit. Aim to consume fruit in the morning (a sprinkle of low-calorie berries at night is okay) unless you are doing high-intensity training in the afternoon. If you are, eat your fruit within 30 minutes before training instead.

Approved beverages

- Water.

- Herbal tea.

- Tea.^

- Coffee.^

- Diet soft drink or cordial.

Note: Drink unlimited water and herbal tea. Any additional beverages need to be worked into overall daily calorie quota.

^If having tea or coffee with milk, use low- or no-fat milk and work into overall calories and no sugar or you can use sugar replacer.

Menu Plans

The foods listed in the menu plan may vary in calorie count and nutritional breakdown according to brands used. Please use this as a general guide. For a more specific guide, consult a calorie counter. If using substitutes make sure they are equal to or less than the protein, carbohydrate, fat and calorie amount of the food you're replacing (and is ideally low GI with no to minimal processing).

Menu plan for women

Meals	Suggestions	Size	Weight	Protein	Carbs	Fat	Calories
	OPTION 1						
	All-bran	¾ cup	45g	6.8	21.5	1.4	151
	OR						
	Oats, rolled (dry weight)	⅓ cup	45g	4.7	27	3.6	172
	OR						
	Goodness Superfoods® P1, D1	⅓ cup	45g	8.7	17.1	4.2	167
	WITH						
	Diet yoghurt^^^	½ tub	100g	3.8	5.4	0.1	40
Breakfast	**OR**						
	Skim or no-fat milk^^^	¾ cup	200ml	7.8	12	0.3	70
	Fat-free soy milk	¾ cup	200ml	7.0	11.6	0.1	76
	ADD (Optional)						
	Mixed berries (average)	½ cup		1	5.6	0.2	35
	OPTION 2						
	3 egg whites			12.5	0	0	45
	Bürgen soy and linseed bread	1 piece	40g	6.4	12	5.6	98
	Low-fat ham	½ packet	50g	7	2	1.4	48

Meals	Suggestions	Size	Weight	Protein	Carbs	Fat	Calories
	CHOOSE FROM						
	Tuna in springwater	1 small tin	95g	13.6	4.6	1.6	87
	Low-fat ham	½ packet	50g	7	2	1.4	48
	Low-fat turkey or sliced chicken	½ packet	50g	14	1	1	50
	Low-fat cottage cheese	½ tub	125g	15.5	5.5	3.3	118
	Low-fat salmon	small tin	95g	20.3	0	8	155
	Chicken breast (raw)	1 medium piece	75g	16.5	0	1.2	79
	ADD						
	Approved salads/ vegetables to fill you up	Unlimited	Unlimited	Trace only	<10 per 100g	Trace only	25 per cup^
	OR						
	Diet yoghurt^^^	1 tub	200g	5.7	8.1	0.2	80
Snack options	**ADD**						
	All-bran	2 dessert spoons	15g	2.2	7	0	50
	OR (approved low GI fruit, 1 piece)						
	Apple	1 medium	150g	0.5	13	0	52
	Orange	1 medium	150g	0.5	13	0	52
	Peach	1 medium	115g	0.5	7	0	40
	Pear	1 medium	150g	0.5	18	0	69
	Plum	1 medium	100g	0.5	8	0	33
	Grapefruit	½		1	5.6	0.1	34
	Strawberries	½ punnet		2.1	3.4	0.1	28
	Blackberries	½ cup	80g	1	7.5	0.2	40
	Blueberries	½ cup	80g	0.2	9	0.1	41
	Raspberries	½ cup	80g	0.8	5.2	0.1	38

Meals	Suggestions	Size	Weight	Protein	Carbs	Fat	Calories
	PROTEIN (choose 1 from)						
	Tuna in springwater	1 small tin	95g	13.6	4.6	1.6	87
	Low-fat ham	1 packet	100g	14	4	2.8	96
	Low-fat turkey or sliced chicken	1 packet	100g	28	2	2	100
	Low-fat cottage cheese	½ tub	125g	15.5	5.5	3.3	118
	Salmon in springwater	1 small tin	100g	20.3	0	8	155
	Chicken breast (raw)	1 piece	100g	22.3	0	1.6	105
	Lean roast beef (packet, sliced)	1 packet	100g	18.7	0.5	2.9	104
	Firm tofu	½ cup	100g	11.7	0	7.2	123
Lunch	**CARBOHYDRATES (choose 1 from)**						
	Bürgen soy and linseed bread	1 piece	40g	6.2	11.5	3	98
	Yam (raw weight)		150g	2.9	21.2	0.2	98
	Long-grain brown rice (cooked)	½ cup	80g	2.3	25.4	0.8	122
	Chickpeas (cooked)	½ cup		5.4	13	1.8	98
	Lentils, all varieties (canned and drained)	½ cup		6.5	13.8	0.7	89
	Beans (mixed, canned and drained)	½ cup		6.4	13.8	0.5	98
	ADD Approved salads/ vegetables to fill you up	Unlimited	Unlimited	Trace only	<10 per 100g	Trace only	25 per cup^
Snack options	Snack options as above **Note:** Make sure you have some form of carbs (no more than 20g total carbs) before high intensity training — for example 1 pear has 18g carbs. If not training, avoid carbs and have a protein snack.						

Meals	Suggestions	Size	Weight	Protein	Carbs	Fat	Calories
	PROTEIN (choose 1 from)						
	Lean sirloin steak (raw)	palm size^^	150g	36.2	0	2.9	173
	Chicken breast (raw)	palm size^^	150g	42.9	0	1.2	186
	Low-fat white fish (raw) eg bassa, cod	palm size^^	150g	23.6	0	2.7	119
	Lean roast beef (baked and sliced)	palm size^^	150g	48.8	0	5	243
Dinner	Extra lean pork loin chops (raw)	palm size^^	150g	33.5	0	3	160
	Lean lamb leg (roasted and sliced)	palm size^^	150g	37.1	0	11	249
	Firm tofu	1 cup	200g	23.4	0	14.4	246
	WITH						
	Unlimited approved salads/vegetables to fill you up	Unlimited	Unlimited	Trace only	<10 per 100g	Trace only	25 per cup^
	Nestlé diet dessert	1 tub	120g	3.2	13	1	75
	OR						
	Nestlé Peter's no added sugar ice-cream	2 scoops	100g	2.8	4.7	2.8	85
	OR						
Dessert	Diet yoghurt^^^	¾ tub	150g	4.4	5.8	0	60
	AND						
	Cottee's diet topping (optional)	2 table spoons					16
	OR						
	Mixed berries	¼ cup		0.5	2.8	0.1	17

Meals	Suggestions	Size	Weight	Protein	Carbs	Fat	Calories
Beverages	Water	1 glass	250ml				0
	Tea, herbal/black/green	1 cup					2
	Black coffee	1 teaspoon					4
Milk	No-fat milk^^^	Dash	20ml				10
	Low-fat soy milk	Dash	20ml				8
	Skim milk^^^	1 cup	250ml	9.3	12.4	0.3	88
	No-fat soy milk	1 cup	250ml	8.8	14.5	0.1	95
Coffee (café)	Skim-milk cappuccino	1 coffee cup		5.7	8.4	0.2	59
	Skim-milk cappuccino (take away)	1 large take away cup					108
	Soy latte (made with light soy milk)	1 coffee cup		5.4	9.9	2.7	87
Soft drink/ cordial	Diet soda (all similar)	1 can	375ml				2
	Diet cordial (mixed)	1 cup	250ml				4
Alcohol*	Spirits (all very similar; consume with soda water or diet soft drink)	shot/nip	30ml				63
	Wine (white)	1 glass	120ml				80
	Wine (red)	1 glass	120ml				80
	Champagne	1 glass	120ml				80
	Beer	1 schooner	450ml				170
		1 can / bottle	375ml				140
	Low-carb beer	1 bottle	375ml				113

^ Approved salad/vegetables can be eaten in unlimited amounts (nobody ever put on weight from eating salad!). All have less than 10 grams carbohydrate per 100 grams, trace only of fat and protein, approximately 25 to 40 calories per 100 grams. Individual calorie amounts for vegetables and salads have not been included. If you want to calculate each individual type, consult a calorie counter or simply add 25 calories per 1 cup (raw) of approved salad/vegetables you have as an average when calculating your total daily calories.

^^ Palm size indicates palm only (not fingers); hand size indicates size of palm as well as fingers.

^^^ If choosing low-fat milk or yoghurt, calorie figures are slightly higher so adjust accordingly.

* Not included in menu plan, work in calories to overall quota if you do consume.

Menu plan for men

Meals	Suggestions	Size	Weight	Protein	Carbs	Fat	Calories
	OPTION 1						
	All-bran	1¼ cup	75g	11	32	3.2	210
	OR						
	Oats, rolled (dry weight)	½ cup	60g	2.5	36	5.4	200
	OR						
	Goodness Superfoods® P1, D1	½ cup	70g	13	25.5	6.3	250
	WITH						
	Diet yoghurt^^^	1 tub	200g	5.7	8.1	0	80
	OR						
Breakfast	Skim or no-fat milk^^^	¾ cup	200ml	7.8	12	0.3	70
	Fat-free soy milk	¾ cup	200ml	7.0	11.6	0.1	96
	ADD (Optional)						
	Mixed berries (average)	½ cup		1.0	5.6	0.2	35
	OPTION 2						
	4 egg whites			16	0	0	60
	Bürgen soy and linseed bread	1 slice	40g	6.2	11.5	3	98
	Low-fat ham	½ packet	50g	7	2	1.4	48
	ADD (optional)						
	Low-fat cheese	1 slice	15g	3.6	0.5	3	36

Meals	Suggestions	Size	Weight	Protein	Carbs	Fat	Calories
	PROTEIN (choose 1 from)						
	Tuna in springwater	1 small tin	95g	13.6	4.6	1.6	87
	Low-fat ham	1 packet	100g	14	4	2.8	96
	Low-fat turkey or sliced chicken	½ packet	50g	14	1	1	50
	Low-fat cottage cheese	½ tub	125g	15.5	5.5	3.3	118
	Low-fat salmon	small tin	95g	20.3	0	8	155
	Chicken breast (raw)	1 large piece	125g	41	0	3.5	145
	ADD						
	Approved salads/vegetables to fill you up						
	OR						
	Diet yoghurt^^^	1 tub	200g	5.7	8.1	0.2	80
Snack options	**ADD**						
	All-bran	2 dessert spoons	15g	2.2	7	0	50
	OR (approved low GI fruit, 1 piece)						
	Apple	1 medium	150g	0.5	13	0	52
	Orange	1 medium	150g	0.5	13	0	52
	Peach	1 medium	115g	0.5	7	0	40
	Pear	1 medium	150g	0.5	18	0	69
	Plum	1 medium	100g	0.5	8	0	33
	Strawberries	½ punnet		2.1	3.4	0.1	28
	Blackberries	½ cup	80g	0.2	10	0	24
	Blueberries	½ cup	80g	0.2	9	0.1	41
	Raspberries	½ cup	80g	0.8	5.2	0.1	38
	Grapefruit	½ (avg.)		1	5.6	0.1	34

Meals	Suggestions	Size	Weight	Protein	Carbs	Fat	Calories
	PROTEIN (choose 1 from)						
	Tuna in springwater	medium tin	190g	27.2	9.2	3.2	174
	Low-fat ham	1½ pack	150g	21	6	4.2	144
	Low-fat turkey or sliced chicken	1½ pack	150g	42	3	2	150
	Low-fat cottage cheese	1 medium tub	250g	31	11	6.6	236
	Salmon in springwater	1 medium tin	190g	40.6	0	16	310
	Chicken breast (raw)	1 piece	150g	35.8	0	1.1	155
	Lean roast beef (packet, sliced)	1½ pack	150g	27.7	0.75	4.5	156
	Firm tofu	1 cup	200g	23.1		14.2	243
Lunch	**CARBOHYDRATES (choose 1 from)**						
	Bürgen soy and linseed bread	2 slices	80g	12.4	23	5.6	197
	Yam (raw weight)		200g	3.8	28.2	0.2	130
	Long grain brown rice (cooked)	¾ cup	120g	3.5	38.2	1.2	183
	Chickpeas (cooked)	¾ cup		8.1	19.5	2.7	147
	Lentils — all varieties (canned and drained)	¾ cup		9.8	20.7	1	133
	Beans (mixed, canned and drained)	¾ cup		9.6	20.7	0.6	147
	ADD						
	Unlimited approved salads/ vegetables to fill you up	unlimited		Trace only	<10 per 100g	Trace only	25 per cup^

Snack options Snack options as above
Note: Make sure you have some form of carbs (no more than 20g total carbs) before high intensity training — for example 1 pear has 18g carbs. If not training, avoid carbs and have a protein snack.

Meals	Suggestions	Size	Weight	Protein	Carbs	Fat	Calories
	PROTEIN (choose 1 from)						
	Lean sirloin steak (raw)	Hand size^^	250g	60	0	7.8	310
	Chicken breast (raw)	Hand size^^	250g	55.8	0	3.6	263
	Low-fat white fish, eg, bassa, cod (raw)	Hand size^^	250g	50	0	2.5	198
Dinner	Lean roast beef (baked and sliced)		250g	81.3	0	8.3	405
	Extra lean pork loin chops (raw)	Hand size^^	250g	55.5	0	4.3	263
	Lean lamb leg (roasted and sliced)		250g	76.5	0	15	445
	Firm tofu	1½ cup	300g	36	0	21.6	381
	WITH						
	Unlimited approved salads/ vegetables to fill you up		Unlimited	Trace only	<10 per 100g	Trace only	25 per cup^
	Nestlé diet dessert	1 tub	120g	3.2	13	1	75
	OR						
	Nestlé Peter's no added sugar ice-cream	2 scoops	100g	2.8	4.7	2.8	85
	OR						
Dessert	Diet yoghurt^^^	¾ tub	150g	4.4	5.8	0	60
	ADD						
	Cottee's diet topping (optional)	2 table spoons					16
	OR						
	Mixed berries (avg.)	¼ cup		0.5	2.8	0.1	17

Meals	Suggestions	Size	Weight	Protein	Carbs	Fat	Calories
Beverages	Water	1 glass	250ml				0
	Tea, herbal/black/green	1 cup					2
	Black coffee	1 teaspoon					4
Milk	No-fat milk	dash	20ml				10
	Low-fat soy milk	dash	20ml				8
	Skim milk	1 cup	250ml	9.3	12.4	0.3	88
	No-fat soy milk	1 cup	250ml	8.8	14.5	0.1	95
Coffee (café)	Skim-milk cappuccino	1 coffee cup		5.7	8.4	0.2	59
	Skim-milk cappuccino (take away)	1 large take-away cup					108
	Soy latte (made with light soy milk)	1 coffee cup		5.4	9.9	2.7	87
Soft drink/ cordial	Diet soda (all similar)	1 can	375ml				2
	Diet cordial (mixed)	1 cup	250ml				4
Alcohol*	Spirits (all very similar; consume with soda water or diet soft drink)	shot/nip	30ml				63
	Wine (white)	1 glass	120ml				80
	Wine (red)	1 glass	120ml				80
	Champagne	1 glass	120ml				80
	Beer	1 schooner	450ml				170
		1 can/ bottle	375ml				140
	Low-carb beer	1 bottle	375ml				113

^ Approved salad/vegetables can be eaten in unlimited amounts (no body ever put on weight from eating salad!). All have less than 10 grams carbohydrate per 100 grams, trace only of fat and protein, approximately 25 to 40 calories per 100 grams. Individual calorie amounts for vegetables and salads have not been included. If you want to calculate each individual type, consult a calorie counter or simply add 25 calories per 1 cup (raw) of approved salad/ vegetables you have as an average when calculating your total daily calories.

^^ Palm size indicates palm only (not fingers); hand size indicates size of palm as well as fingers.

^^^ If choosing low-fat milk or yoghurt, calorie figures are slightly higher so adjust accordingly.

* Not included in menu plan, work in calories to overall quota if you do consume.

Sample menu plans

Below are some examples of how to put together a day's worth of eating using the menu plans (beverages not included in these samples).

Sample Menu Plan — Women

Meal	Sample Day 1	Sample Day 2
Breakfast	⅓ cup oats with ¾ cup no fat milk + ½ cup mixed berries	Egg white omelette made with 3 egg whites, mushroom (or vegetable of your choice from allowed list) cooked in non-stick pan
Snack	1 orange	1 apple
Lunch	Quick chicken salad: 100 grams of sliced chicken + Cos lettuce and rocket leaves + 150 grams (raw weight) of chopped baked sweet potato (dry baked) + ½ sliced red capsicum + Splash of balsamic vinegar	1 piece of soy and linseed bread cut into squares, dipped into 125 grams of low-fat cottage cheese + 2 cups of mixed salad with low-fat dressing
Snack	Carrot and celery sticks dipped in ½ tub low-fat cottage cheese	Diet yoghurt plus sprinkle All-bran
Dinner	Baked fish and vegetables: 150 grams (raw weight) white fish wrapped in foil with fresh herbs, squeeze of lemon juice and dried chilli (optional) + ¼ eggplant, 1 small zucchini, 1 small red onion sprayed with oil spray and baked	Chicken stir-fry: Use a non stick pan or use spray oil to stir-fry: 1 garlic clove, ½ chopped onion, 150 grams (raw weight) chicken breast, sliced green capsicum, bok choy, broccoli florets, green beans + Splash low sodium soy sauce (optional)
Dessert (optional)	None	2 scoops no-added-sugar ice-cream + sprinkle mixed berries

Sample Menu Plan — Men

Meal	Sample Day 1	Sample Day 2
Breakfast	4 egg whites scrambled in non-stick pan + low-fat ham + low-fat cheese on top of soy linseed toast, grilled	1¼ cup All-bran + ¾ cup fat free soy milk + ½ cup mixed berries
Snack	1 peach	1 pear
Lunch	1 medium tin salmon in springwater + ¾ cup four bean mix + chopped shallots + sliced celery + splash balsamic vinegar + cracked black pepper	Ham and salad sandwich: 2 slices of soy and linseed bread + 150g low-fat ham or turkey + lettuce, tomato, shredded carrot and onion
Snack	½ packet low-fat ham rolled up into 'cigars' using ¼ tub low-fat cottage cheese + chopped cucumber	1 tin of flavoured (such as lemon and cracked pepper) tuna in springwater
Dinner	250g (raw weight) lean sirloin steak cooked in non-stick pan with 1 chopped onion and sliced mushrooms dry-fried and spooned on top of steak + Mixed salad with low-fat dressing	250g (roasted and sliced) lean lamb leg with rosemary, parsley, garlic and lemon + steamed green beans and snow peas + grilled asparagus
Dessert (optional)	¾ tub diet yoghurt + sprinkle of mixed berries	None

PART 3: SHAPE UP!

Now you've got your eating on track, it's time to hit the exercise track. Get ready to walk, run, jump, sprint, pedal, push, pull, lift, skip, grunt, stretch — and sweat! You're going to hit it hard with a mixture of circuit training and resistance training to totally reshape your body, along with cardio training to burn up loads of calories and fat. There's a training program suited to every level of fitness. All you have to do is make a start and build up to a fitter, stronger, slimmer and healthier you! Remember, results and satisfaction come from doing the hard yards in your training and building strength — physically and mentally! Let's get to it.

Chapter 7:
The Heads UP on Fitness for Fat Loss

When it comes to working out for weight loss it's not so much what you do but rather the *quality* and *quantity* of what you do. The overall objective is to burn as many calories through activity as possible and build up some muscle tone so as you lose weight you look trim, toned and terrific! People are always looking for 'the best' exercise. The simple answer is there isn't one. You simply need to start moving more, then as your body adapts to moving more, you need to move faster and for longer!

Let's kick off with some convincing reasons to move your body.

Why exercise is king (or queen!)

There's no doubt about it: exercise is imperative for a fit, vital and trim body, and a better quality of life. Here are some of the pay-offs of regular physical activity.

- Look better in your clothes.

- Healthy blood pressure.

- Ease of living — makes everyday things like bending over to shave your legs, tie shoelaces or picking up the shopping possible.

- Cholesterol management (boosts good cholesterol and decreases bad cholesterol).

- Better breathing capacity.

- Combats chronic disease such as stroke, Type 2 diabetes, heart disease and some types of cancers.

- Reduced risk of overweight- and obesity-related health conditions such as sleep apnoea.

- Boosts bone density and offsets osteoporosis.

- Maintains muscle mass and metabolism.

- Builds strength and stamina.

- Reduces stress levels and puts you in a good mood.

- Assists in the prevention and treatment of mental illness such as depression and anxiety disorders.

- Increased flexibility, mobility, coordination and body balance.

- Improved insulin sensitivity (important for the prevention and management of Metabolic Syndrome and Type 2 diabetes).

- Anti-ageing by preventing loss of muscle mass, which contributes to sagging skin, and keeps ageing joints mobile.

- Weight management and body fat reduction.

- Ramps up calorie expenditure — even when you are at rest.

- Better sleep and improved libido.

- More energy and stamina.

- Strengthens self-esteem.

> Did you know that physical inactivity ranks second only to tobacco smoking in terms of disease prevention in Australia?

How exercise helps you lose weight

While diet is the main deciding factor in whether or not you'll drop weight (you can exercise as much as you like but if you don't eat right you won't lose much weight), exercise is critical not only for the health and lifestyle reasons listed above, but to assist and accelerate the weight-loss process. Exercise works to help you lose weight in three key ways.

1. It burns calories and fat.

The key to successful fat loss is making a calorie deficit (as we talked about in Part 2: Eat Up!) — the bigger the deficit the bigger and faster the weight loss. Exercise helps to ramp up your calorie expenditure both during a workout and afterwards. You see, post exercise, your metabolism remains raised, especially after a strenuous workout where the 'after burn' effect is enhanced. This effect is known as Excess Post-Exercise Oxygen Consumption (EPOC), which, in a layperson's terms, refers to the excess energy (calories) used to restore the body to its resting, pre-exercise state and make adaptations from the exertion. When you're trying to burn as many calories as possible, you can see why this is a huge bonus!

2. It builds lean muscle tissue.

In a nutshell, people with a higher muscle mass naturally have higher metabolisms so they burn more calories in a day. Also, after a resistance workout the increased activity of your muscles rebuilding and repairing actually burns calories so your fat burning rate remains raised for hours after you've left the gym!

Combine high-intensity cardio with resistance training and you will burn fat — day and night!

3. It makes you feel better.

When you feel good about your efforts to exercise you're more likely to make healthy food choices so as not to 'spoil' your hard work. Your self-esteem and positive outlook also increases, influencing the health and fitness choices you make.

Okay, now that we've jogged your memory as to why you need to get your butt into gear, let's look at the type of movement you need to do.

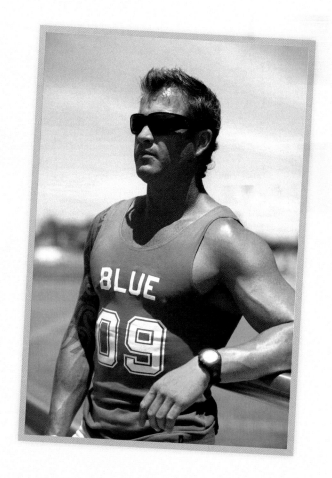

Four ways to move

There are three staples to building a complete fitness program, known as the three S's of fitness: stamina, strength, suppleness. You achieve these staples by doing **cardio**, **resistance**, and **flexibility** training. For further health and weight-loss benefits, there's a fourth activity you need to include: **incidental activity**.

1. Get your activity levels up — incidental activity

One of the best and simplest ways to begin is to simply move more in your day-to-day life. For most, if coupled with a change in diet, this will be enough to start dropping weight immediately. How inspiring is that!

Once you build more incidental activity — the kind of everyday activity you do outside of planned exercise sessions such as housework, taking the dog for a walk and gardening — you'll not only set your weight loss off to a good start but you'll ingrain an activity habit into your life. This will ensure you keep up a healthy lifestyle and complement your weight loss through extra calorie burning once you're into a regular exercise program. Some ways to ramp up your day-to-day activity levels include:

- Gardening, weeding, and digging.

- Mowing the lawn (I still have an old-school lawn mower; no engine, just Ponton power!).

- Take a walk break instead of a coffee or cigarette break.

- Walk instead of taking public transport or driving.

- Get off the train or bus a few stops earlier and hike the rest of the way.

- Always take the stairs instead of the lift and escalator.

- Play with your kids: jump on the trampoline, shoot hoops in the yard, go for a ride together, kick a footy down the local park (they'll love you for it and all the while you're burning calories).

- Hand deliver your messages at work instead of emailing them.

- Grab your low-fat coffee takeaway and meet your friend for a walk-and-talk instead of sitting in at the café.

- Ditch technology: get up off the couch to change the channel, wash the dishes, hang your clothes out, sweep the floors.

- Clean and wash the car yourself.

- Do the handiwork around the house such as sanding and painting, instead of sourcing it out.

- Take the furthest parking spot from the entrance (you'll save yourself the stress too).

- Walk the dog or a neighbour's dog.

- Walk the kids to school instead of driving them.

- Plan active weekends such as a picnic in the park and a game of cricket; horse riding; a day at the beach swimming, surfing, Frisbee-throwing and playing beach volleyball; bushwalks; and so on.

Get your steps up!

A simple way to keep your daily activity levels in check is to wear a pedometer — a tiny device that attaches to your belt or pants that detects movement and clocks up the amount of steps you take in a day. Health authorities recommend at least 10,000 steps a day. This is a great place to start building up and maintaining your incidental activity. Don't think that doing a sweat session at the gym provides you with a permission slip to sit at your desk all day and plonk your feet up on the couch when you get home. An all-round active lifestyle is a must for continued calorie expenditure and long-term health.

2. Get your heart rate up — cardio

The next step up from increased incidental activity is the huff-and-puff kind — cardio (also called aerobic exercise). This type of activity involves the use of large muscle groups, moving in a repetitive rhythmic action over a sustained period of time. It increases your heart and breathing rate, making you puff!

Cardio builds cardiovascular fitness (endurance), increases stamina, keeps your heart and lungs healthy, boosts oxygen flow around the body, tops up happy and stress-reducing hormones and brain neurotransmitters such as endorphins and serotonin, and burns up calories and fat. Aerobic literally means 'with oxygen' and utilises fat and carbohydrates as the primary source of fuel to be converted into the energy required to perform exercise for extended periods.

Common forms of cardio include walking, running, swimming, cycling, boxing, aerobics-based exercise classes, dancing, circuit training and many sports such as basketball, football, tennis, and so on.

In terms of using swimming as a form of cardio, it's best kept for leisure, fun, and injury rehabilitation. Although it's a lovely form of cardio with many health benefits, it just doesn't cut it in the calorie and fat-burning stakes because of its non-weight bearing nature. This makes it great for groups that need to take pressure off of the joints when exercising — injury rehabilitation, post-exercise recovery, pregnancy, arthritis, obesity, and so on — but weight bearing exercise works best for weight loss. If you are using the pool to work out, get the most calorie burn for your splash by including high intensity moves such as sprinting laps, deep water running or using water resistance devices such as floating medicine balls and aqua dumbbells.

3. Firm up — resistance training

We tighten, tone, strengthen and build up our muscles through resistance training. Simply put, if cardio is huff-and-puff exercise, resistance training is lift-and-grunt exercise. Think of any exercise where you have to 'muscle' a load. This load can come in many forms such as your bodyweight, a dumbbell or barbell, machine weights, a medicine ball or a resistance band.

Resistance training (also called strength or weight training) not only gives your body a better overall look, it builds lean muscle which is your best weapon to keep burning calories and fat all day, strengthens bones to ward off osteoporosis, triggers the anti-ageing human growth hormone (HGH), improves exercise performance, facilitates sport-specific strength and power, strengthens muscles to help you handle anaerobic training like sprints, and assists in better body balance and posture — so you feel stronger, leaner, younger and better!

Common forms of resistance training include lifting weights, circuit training, body-weight exercises like push-ups and sit-ups, climbing stairs, using a resistance band, a Pump class at the gym, and so on.

4. Loosen up — flexibility training

Loosening up is just as important as firming up. Tight, tense muscles cause a host of problems such as soreness and pain which makes it hard to back up for multiple training sessions, injury, postural imbalances, stress and tension caused by energy blockages in the body, reduced

range of motion for exercise and everyday activities, and not being able to spring out of bed every morning.

Use it or lose it

There's a reason people get slower, fatter, less stronger and more prone to injury and illness — because they don't use their muscles enough. Muscle mass reaches its peak in most people around their mid twenties, then declines in their thirties and forties, with the rate of loss accelerating even more once they hit 50. To put it plainly: lack of use will cause your muscles to slowly waste away and quite literally shrivel up and die! Although aerobic exercise like walking, swimming and running is good for you, this type of exercise just won't cut it in terms of maintaining your muscle mass and strength. Your muscles are the powerhouses of your body and if you want to stay physically young and healthy, and be able to keep doing everyday things you take for granted like open a stubborn jar lid or piggyback your kids, you've got to use those muscles!

To loosen up we need to s-t-r-e-t-c-h! (That feels better already, doesn't it?) Stretching can be done separately (called flexibility training) or as part of your workout in the warm up and cool down.

Regular stretching helps to prevent and rehabilitate injury, reduce stress, prepare your body for a workout, rid your muscles of lactic acid post-workout, improve circulation, and give you a healthier posture, which all combine towards helping you feel more relaxed, energetic, youthful and taller!

There are two types of stretching: static and dynamic. Static stretching is the most common form and involves taking your muscle to an end point of stretch and holding for a set amount of seconds such as placing your leg on a chair to stretch your hamstring. Dynamic stretching involves stretching and mobilising the muscles through range-of-motion type stretches such as leg swings or shoulder rolls.

Common forms of flexibility training include stretching, stretching with aids such as straps and Swiss balls, yoga and body balance classes.

After neglecting stretching for 20 years, at the ripe old age of 37 I finally realised just how important an appropriate stretch routine is and started Power Living Yoga. If you're thinking 'om's and linen trousers, think again. It's a full-on rhythmic and dynamic form of yoga that's not only enhanced my flexibility, core strength and focus but also facilitated a newfound inward clarity. (Oh... and a newfound humility, too, as the entire class audibly delighted in my discomfort and lame flexibility!)

Muscle make-up

Did you know that you use different muscle fibres when you jump than walk? Fast twitch (Type II; anaerobic) muscle fibres are the ones you use to do fast, powerful, more explosive movements like jump, sprint or lift something heavy. Slow twitch (Type I; aerobic) muscle fibres are used to do slower, steady, more sustained movements like going for a walk or jog.

Everyone has a different ratio of these muscle fibres. Those with slow twitch (endurance) fibres tend to be naturals (the born-to-run types) at endurance events such as running, swimming, cycling and triathlons. Those with a higher ratio of fast twitch (power) muscle fibres tend to be better at shorter, faster events like sprinting, weight and power lifting, and long jump.

Because these muscle fibres decline with age, it's important to pay attention to both types of fibres in your training. Lifting a heavy weight for low repetitions and doing plyometrics and sprints stimulates growth and strength in your fast twitch/ anaerobic fibres. Lifting a low weight for high repetitions and doing steady, continuous cardio hits your slow twitch/aerobic fibres.

Including both anaerobic and aerobic styles of training produces superior results for strength, power, speed and fat burning — you'll cover all bases and you'll be well on your way to some kick-ass results!

Top training methods

After being in the fitness industry for 20 years, I've come to know what really works to strip fat and boost fitness — fast! Here are my top training methods for super fitness and weight loss.

The calories burnt quoted for each form of exercise are a general guide only. Calories burnt vary greatly according to age, weight, gender, muscle mass, fitness level and intensity (how hard you go!). Figures quoted (marked with an asterisk) are based on an average 85 kilogram male. For a general indication of the calories burnt according to your gender and weight you can use an online calculator or calorie expenditure chart, but the only way to guarantee how many calories you are burning is to use a heart-rate monitor which measures your exact calorie expenditure when you exercise.

Running

The best part about running is that you don't require any experience or equipment to do it. Just throw on a good pair of running shoes and away you go! Running rates high in the calorie-burning stakes making it an easy and effective way to drop fat. You can run in the gym on a treadmill, around your neighbourhood or local park or through inspiring scenery such as the beach or bush.

Burn it up: Slow jogging uses an average of 300–500* calories per hour. Running uses an average of 700–900* calories per hour.

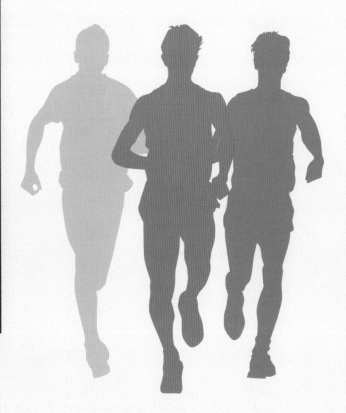

Anyone for a run?

Anyone can run (provided you don't have any pre-diagnosed medical or physical conditions), no matter how de-conditioned or overweight you are. It's been proven year after year on *The Biggest Loser* with all contestants being able to do some form of running once they leave the house. In series 5, in just 12 weeks of dramatically, physically and mentally transforming 11 morbidly obese people, they completed a full marathon!

Here's how.

Do this program 2–3 times a week for 20–45 minutes.

- Start with a walk/jog interval, for example, use street-light posts as markers and walk one light post, then jog one light post; or use a stopwatch and time yourself on a treadmill or outdoors and walk for 30 seconds, then jog for 30 seconds.

- Gradually build up your speed and total workout time (this may be as low 10 minutes to start with).

- Next increase your work intervals and decrease the rest intervals, for example, walk one light post, run two light posts or walk/rest 30 seconds, jog 1 minute.

- Keep bridging the gap by having less time for the walk/rest interval, more time for the run interval until you're running continuously for longer bouts, working up to being able to run for 20 plus minutes without stopping.

Now, that you are officially a runner, why not try your first fun run? Here are some tips:

Get yourself a correctly fitted running shoe

Correct footwear is one of the most important things to address when commencing a training/running program to avoid an injury. Get a running shoe, not a cross trainer. Not only should your shoe be correctly fitted you must chose the correct type of runner. Do you roll in or roll out? This can be done professionally at Athlete's Foot or a specific runner's shop.

Prepare

Give yourself enough time to build up the volume of your training.

Beginner: It should take you at least 6 weeks to gradually increase the amount of kilometres you run each week. Try running or even walk/run 2–4 kilometres, 2–3 times in the first week. Each week increase the distance you run by 2 kilometres. At the end of 6 weeks you will be running 12 kilometres and should be just about race ready.

Intermediate and advanced runners:
You will benefit most from a combination of shorter fast runs, hill sprints and longer distances (about 25–30 per cent less than race distance) at a slightly higher intensity than that at which you usually run.

Training specificity

If you want to become a better runner you must run. Sounds simple but a lot of people make this very mistake. Make the event you are going to compete in the focus of your training schedule.

Structure active recovery

Use cross-training as structured recovery, for example, a cycle class which is non-impact will allow your legs and joints to recover and still aid your overall fitness. Remember, it is only a synergist (assistant) to your overall conditioning and actual running.

Training intensity

Gradually increase your training intensity. You can do this in one of three ways.

1. Set a course and each time aim to run that course a little faster.

2. Gradually increase the distance you run each week.

3. Try using a heart-rate monitor. It is the ultimate tool for checking training intensity. You can run at a pre-set heart rate, say 150 bpm (beats per minute) for 30 minutes, and each week increase it to say 170 bpm for 30 minutes.

Check technique

To get the most out of your running, you need to hold yourself tall while you run. This can be tough if you're absolutely stuffed! But if you're bent over, your airways and lungs are squashed, giving you less surface space to suck air in. By keeping your postural muscles erect, your core strong and switched on, as well as good integrity through your hips and torso, you'll get a better running performance and be able to run a lot more efficiently and for longer.

Enjoy all aspects

Most of all, enjoy every aspect of training, preparation, and, of course, race day. During the race take time to look around, enjoy the challenge, embrace the emotional rollercoaster you will go on, believe in yourself, and don't quit. Push through the different psychological and physical barriers you encounter. You will learn a lot about just how strong you are mentally. Finally the finish: enjoy running across the line, check the clock, note your time and hold onto the empowering feeling of having completed your goal. Then, gear up to beat your time next run!

Indoor cycling

I've been a cycle instructor for many years. This awesome cycle-to-music class is done on specially designed, stationary bikes set up in an indoor cycling studio usually within a gym. It's a highly motivating class that uses visualisation, intervals, sprints and 'hill climbs' to pedal away the pounds! Also super for toning the thighs and butt.

Burn it up: If you push yourself hard (the harder and faster the better!) in an indoor cycling class, you can expect to burn 750–900* calories an hour.

Boxing

If you're looking for a good old-fashioned gut-busting session, you can't go past boxing. Boxers are among the fittest and toughest athletes in the world. The high-intensity nature of going a round (or mimicking it through boxing-based workouts) means you burn loads of calories and work up a serious sweat! Boxing will also improve your cardio fitness, power, balance, coordination, strength, agility and speed. On top of these physical benefits it does wonders for stress relief, building self-confidence, self-defence skills and giving you a feeling of empowerment.

You don't need to be in the ring to benefit from boxing. You can set up a bag in your garage, box with a training partner or personal trainer with focus pads and mitts, do a boxing-based circuit class, and even try kickboxing within any of these boxing formats.

Burn it up: A boxing-style workout uses an average of 500–800* calories per hour. Step into the ring and watch that number skyrocket! I've burned over 600* calories in 40 minutes of sparring.

Skip to it

Skipping is a secret training weapon used by all boxers as part of their training routine. It's super for calorie burning (a 10-minute skip session can burn up to 120 calories), coordination, speed, balance and agility — it's also fun! Skipping can be tough on your joints and lower back if you're overweight so work up to it, doing small bouts of jumping as part of an overall circuit, with plenty of rest breaks in between.

Weight training

Many people focus on cardio when trying to lose weight, but adding weight training to the mix kicks the process along by way of building metabolism-making muscle and giving your body a more toned look as you lose the fat.

When it comes to lifting weights many women baulk at the fear of putting on bulk! Ladies, listen up: it's very, very, very hard to put on 'manly' muscle size. You need testosterone and hours in the weights room in order to put on bulk. Women don't have these high levels of testosterone and as a general rule weight training tones, strengthens and shapes the female body rather than making it bigger and bulkier.

Burn it up: A light weight-training session uses around 200* calories an hour; a strenuous weight-training session uses around 400* calories an hour.

> Ladies, don't baulk at the thought of bulk. Testosterone makes you seven to ten times more likely to gain muscle and females don't have high levels of testosterone.

Circuit training

Circuit training simply means moving from one exercise to the next, doing the exercise for a set of repetitions or period of time before moving to the next exercise station, with little to no rest in between exercises.

There are endless circuit combinations that can be done with or without equipment: using weight machines or free weights, outdoors using logs and park benches, at home using chairs, coffee tables and resistance bands, or as a circuit class. There are also weight-training circuits, cardio mixed with resistance-training circuits and circuits that shift between different body parts.

Doing weights in a circuit style increases the calorie expenditure of a standard weights workout. And doing circuits which switch between upper body, lower body and abdominal exercises work to shunt the blood around to opposite ends of the body (called Peripheral Heart Action — see Phase 3 in the Hard'n Up Training Program on 186) making your body work harder, giving you more burn for your buck!

Burn it up: High-intensity circuit training with minimal rest periods uses an average of 560–800* calories per hour.

Interval training

Interval training is a powerful training tool for novice and advanced exercises. It simply involves shifting between bursts of more intense and less intense intervals, such as cycling at a steady rate on a stationary bike, sprinting for a song track, then pedalling at a steady pace again to recover, before sprinting again. By alternating between different work levels, you score a bigger overall burn than doing continuous cardio at the same intensity. For example, a 45-minute walk with hills and stairs (higher-intensity intervals) scattered throughout will burn loads more calories than a 45-minute walk on a flat walk path.

Another pay-off of interval training is that it improves your fitness much faster by training at higher intensities.

You can apply an interval-training format to walking, running, cycling, boxing and using cardio equipment in the gym.

Burn it up: The calories used in an interval-training workout will vary, depending on the format of the program and the type of exercise you do, but you can expect to burn up to 600–900* calories per hour during high-intensity interval training.

Many studies confirm that interval training, including sprint intervals, burns the most fat and gets the best fitness and weight-loss results. One Aussie study found that a 20-minute workout on a stationary bike, including 8-second sprint intervals followed by 12 seconds recovery pedalling at a slow pace, produced greater fat loss, specifically from the thighs and waist.

Exercise classes

Exercise classes are an affordable way to get access to a similar source of motivation and guidance to group personal training. When you do an exercise class, the upbeat energy is shared among the group, making it hard to slow down and back off when you feel tired or if you have a tendency to do so when working out on your own. You'll be swept up in the power and passion, and be pushed to new limits. And the best part? Because you're having fun and you're stimulated, the class will be over before you know it (sure beats counting down monotonous minutes on a treadmill!). The regularity of committing to a class timetable also helps you stick to an exercise routine.

Aside from indoor cycling, my favourite exercise classes are body attack, Hi-NRG aerobics, basic training, boot camp, and cross fit.

Cross Fit is a high intensity military style workout that combines elements of gymnastics, power lifting and athletics. It's a very effective and efficient way to train. Make sure you go to a registered Cross Fit Centre, as you will need a lot of coaching on technique and form before you are ready to compete (even if you're an experienced trainer). Suited to hardcore participants!

Burn it up: Calories burned vary according to the type of class, but for high-intensity aerobics-based classes expect to burn upwards of 500–800* calories an hour. (I've burned 970* calories teaching a one-hour body attack class!)

At the end of the day, while these training methods have extra benefits for losing weight, any exercise done regularly and at a good intensity will help you lose weight — providing you eat right.

Shannan's workout routine

I take keeping fit and healthy very seriously. I train most days of the week and am very passionate about running and boxing, among other things. Here's what a typical week's worth of training looks like, when I'm not living and eating with *The Biggest Loser* contestants.

Monday

am

Weight training: chest and triceps x 45 minutes plus stretch

pm

1 hour teaching a spin class or Hi-NRG aerobics

Tuesday

am

Boxing x 1 hour plus weight training: back and biceps

pm

Rugby League training (I still train the local A-grade side, 'The Harbord Valley Spartans'.)

Wednesday

am

Mixed martial arts training x 1 hour

Lunch

Power Living Yoga x 1 hour

Thursday

am

Boxing x 1 hour plus weight training: shoulders and legs

Friday

am

Mixed martial arts training or 5-10 kilometre run

Lunch

Power Living Yoga x 1 hour

Saturday

am

Boxing x 2 hours

pm

Weight Training: total body x 30 minutes

Sunday

Rest or body attack class

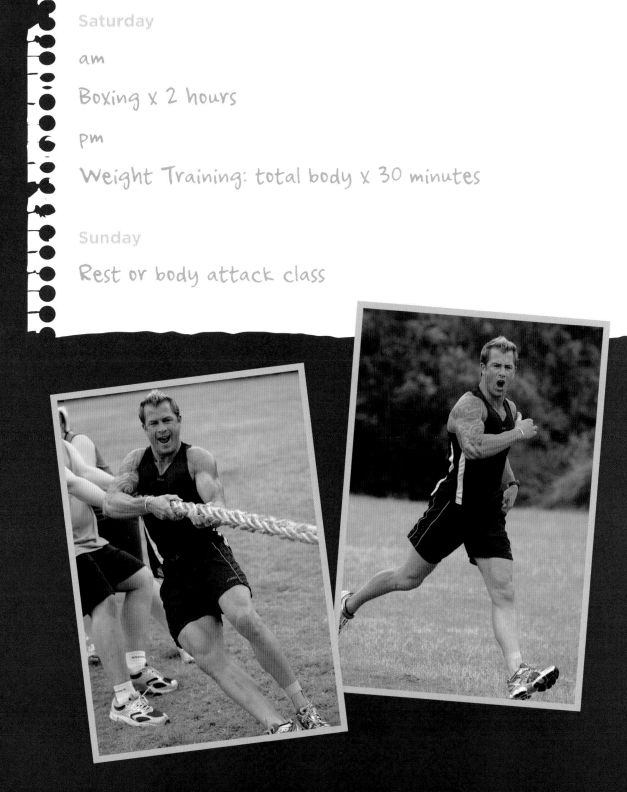

THE HEADS UP ON FITNESS FOR FAT LOSS

Chapter 8:
Rip it UP — The Hard'n Up Training Program

When it comes to working out, the harder you push, the more you do, the faster you'll see results. You and you alone reap the rewards of your own diligence.

Time to roll your sleeves up, get to work and hard'n up!

Get a check-up

Before even attempting any training program it is essential that you get a full check-up from your doctor. The doctor should issue you with a clearance to commence training and offer advice on your individual limits and exercise contraindications specific to you. Seek advice from a fitness professional to ensure safety, efficiency and correct technique. Listen to your body (stop if you are feeling dizzy, sick or faint) and never compromise your health or safety for that extra rep or metre.

Training is a metaphor for life. If you're a quitter, too soft, an exaggerator, a liar, or unreliable, it will be expressed in the way you train. Set goals, focus, work hard, be disciplined and you'll reap the respect and results you deserve.

About the training program — 8 training philosophies

The Hard'n Up Training Program has been developed over many years in the fitness industry. These programs work! They are tried and tested for fast and effective fat loss and muscle toning. My training programs have helped many overweight people — including *The Biggest Loser* contestants — turn their lives around, reshape their bodies and drop staggering amounts of weight.

The training program is based on eight training philosophies.

1. Get to a gym.

2. Move with a mate.

3. Make it count.

4. Find exercise you enjoy.

5. You get out what you put in.

6. Combine resistance and cardio.

7. Set new personal bests — increase intensity.

8. Results come from commitment and consistency.

1. Get to a gym

I'm a big believer in going to a gym because it offers you so many things you can't get from your training when doing it at home alone. A gym is packed with specialised equipment, a diverse range of exercise classes for all fitness and coordination levels, and gives you direct access to trained professionals. Plus, the gym provides a focused space where you don't have any interruptions to take you away from your workout — such as work, phone calls, or the kids — giving you the chance to put everything aside and to concentrate on you!

Many are faced with apprehensive thoughts when thinking about joining a gym. (Heard the line, 'I gotta get fit to go to the gym, gotta go to the gym to get fit' before?) Some of these apprehensive thoughts might be: 'I don't know how to use the equipment so I'll be embarrassed'; 'I'll be out of place among all those slim, fit bodies'; 'I won't know what to do'; 'People will stare at me'. If these self-defeating thoughts sound familiar and you're afraid of going to the gym, this is a time where you have to hard'n up, face your fears and get in there. You'll be surprised at how much the fitness instructors and other members are there to help, support and encourage you — if not, shop around for a more suitable gym.

When finding a gym, do your homework and find the right fit. If money is an issue, local YMCA, community-run, or RSL gyms can be a much cheaper option or find a gym where you can pay by the month.

2. Move with a mate

Training with someone — be it a training partner or personal trainer — makes you accountable (people are less likely to let someone else down by not turning up to a planned and/or paid session than letting themselves down), and pushes you to work much harder than you would if exercising on your own.

Having your own personal trainer used to be a luxury, reserved only for the rich and famous. Now, thanks to a burgeoning industry, there are loads of great and affordable personal trainers in most areas of the country. And if you think you can't afford a personal trainer, look into group personal training (where the cost is shared between members of the group). Group sessions start at around $15 per person (the more people in the group, the less cost per person). Personal training can be done in the home, gym, at work, in a personal training studio or anywhere in the great outdoors.

Hooking up with a workout buddy is a great alternative if a personal trainer or gym membership is not in the budget at the moment. It's also a great complement to your training program even if you do go to the gym or have a trainer. The best places to find a training partner include family, work colleagues, mother's group, neighbours, friends and school parents.

As the trainer on *The Biggest Loser*, and with a lifetime of fitness experience, I still need a trainer – three, actually! I have two boxing trainers and a mixed martial arts trainer (each one pushes me to my potential, way beyond what I perceive as my limit, and all delight in the regular occurrences of me heaving my guts up over the ropes or in the cage!). I also have an awesome training partner, my mate Shayne, of 18 years (during this time you could count on one hand the number of sessions one of us has missed!). Having a tough, committed, like-minded training partner, as well as a 'trainer's trainer' is essential to keep pushing my mind and body and learn new things.

Find a friend in fitness

Having someone to push, teach, guide, support and encourage you is a huge help. Here's a guide to finding your perfect fitness match.

Gym

Perks	What to look for in a gym
• Experienced and qualified instructors to teach you.	• Good customer service!
• Social and supportive element of the other members.	• Fitness assessment (including a pre-screening questionnaire) prior to commencement of your gym program.
• Specialises in delivering results.	• Fitness programming.
• All the proper tools you need to transform your body at your disposal which maximises training efficiency.	• Regular check-up on your progress, fitness re-assessments, and program updates.
• Use of specialised weight machines and equipment you don't normally have access to at home.	• Friendly, professional staff.
• Wide variety of exercise classes on offer — everything from dance based classes to boxing to yoga.	• Has qualified fitness instructors, manning the floor at all times, to watch your technique and answer your questions.
• Access to fitness assessments and re-assessments.	• The right fit: there are many gym styles on offer with different points of focus, such as boxing gyms, a diverse fitness club with a wide range of classes and equipment, a body-builders gym, an all-female fitness centre, and so on.
• Experts on hand to answer your burning fitness questions.	• A crèche, if needed.
	• Has an exit option. Make sure you read the fine print on the contract and can opt out without heavy financial penalty should you get injured or find that the gym isn't up to scratch.

Personal trainer

Perks	What to look for in a personal trainer
• Maximises the efficiency of your workout.	• Do you want male or female?
• Someone to be accountable to, whether to drag you out of bed or make you pay (in both senses of the word: physically and financially!) for missing a workout.	• Must be fully qualified and insured.
	• Proven track record: experience and results are your best bet in finding a good trainer.
• Individual attention and expertise to teach you the ropes.	• Any specialities that suit your goals — such as pre- and post-natal, weight loss, injury rehabilitation, boxing, sport specific, body balance and core stability, added yoga or Pilates qualifications.
• Can tailor a program specific to your goals and lifestyle.	
• Injury rehabilitation programming (for advanced cases, a qualified exercise physiologist may be required).	• A good listener who responds to your needs, goals, and questions. You pay a personal trainer for results; if you're not getting the results you want, get a new trainer (you wouldn't keep going to the same hairdresser or mechanic if you weren't getting the results you pay for).
• Ensures correct exercise technique, which can be translated to safe exercising at home on your own.	
• Regular monitoring of your progress and weight loss.	
• Basic dietary, health, and lifestyle advice.	

Training partner

Perks	What to look for in a training partner
• Doesn't cost anything.	• Positive and motivated.
• You can egg each other on.	• Like-minded.
• Spot one another and watch technique.	• Weight training experience if you're a novice and need someone to show you the ropes.
• You can teach each other exercises and training tips.	• Ideally of a similar fitness level for cardio workouts so one person doesn't get held back (although circuit training can cater for all fitness levels).
• Help each other stay on the exercise straight-and-narrow when the other feels like slacking off or skipping a workout.	

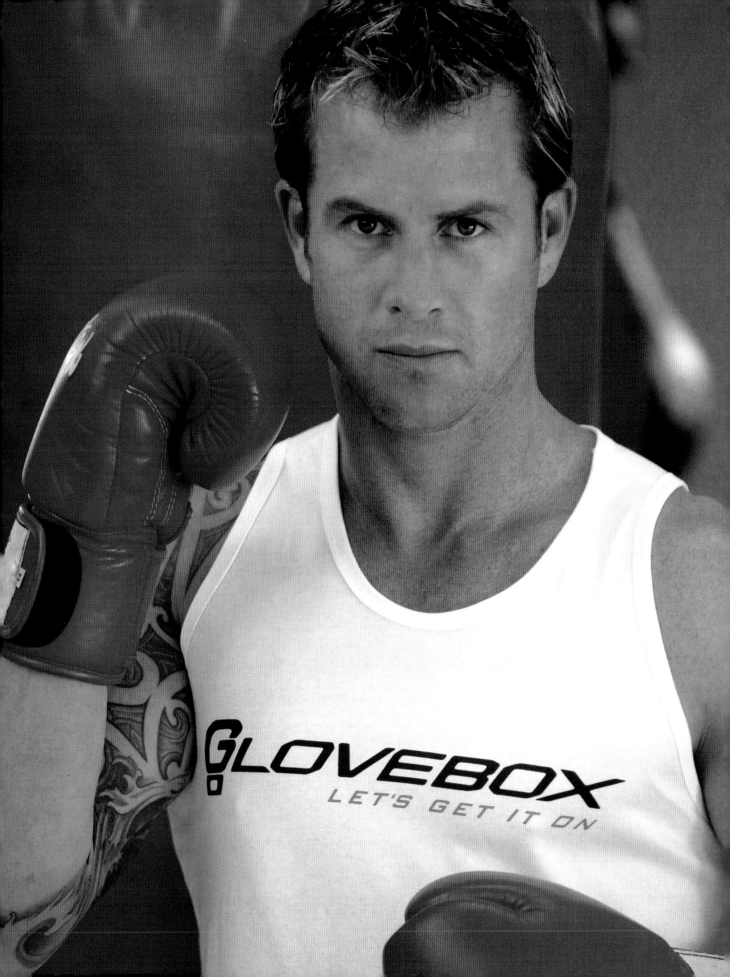

3. Make it count

Whether you've got a little or a lot of time to exercise, you want to get the most for your money. The failproof rule is: if you've only got 10 minutes, go as hard and fast as you can (anaerobic); if you can set aside an hour, roll back the intensity and crank up the volume and go slower for longer (aerobic). The key is to cut the excuses and make the most of *any* opportunity you have to move/train.

4. Find exercise you enjoy

Experiment with different training modalities. Exercise doesn't have to be a hard slog all of the time. In fact, the more enjoyment you derive from exercise the more chance you have of making it a part of your lifestyle for good. Search around for ways to exercise that you like. This may be a sport, a new exercise class, working out to music or training in a group for the social and motivating aspect. Some people find their exercise niche faster than others but there's something for everyone out there in the field of fitness, so keep searching! Whatever you choose to do, remember — it's training hard at it that matters the most!

5. Combine resistance and cardio

If you're after that lean, ripped, toned body you need to combine weights (to tone up) with cardio (to burn fat). Combining both training methods will strip the 'puffy' layer covering your muscles giving you that toned look you long for. That's why resistance and cardio training complement one another and also pack a powerful calorie-burning combination.

6. You get out what you put in

When it comes to a workout you get out of it what you put into it — the harder you work, the more you burn. You may even feel like vomiting; this is a common occurrence when you're really unfit or when you push yourself to the max — providing you have supervision, this is ok. Hard'n up!

Pain is just weakness leaving the body.

Burn baby

The aerobic system (with oxygen) is the system we rely on for everyday living. Aerobic energy requires the use of carbohydrates and fats. These are broken down in a complex chemical process to form ATP (adenosine tri phosphate) and carbon dioxide, heat and water as by-products. It is the system that is dominant in long distance events. But switch to a short, fast, explosive, more intense activity, if there's not enough oxygen to meet the increased demands of the new workload, your body calls on another system of energy known as the anaerobic system (without oxygen). There are two chains under the anaerobic system: the ATP–PC cycle, which provides energy for short explosive activities such as sprinting, pushing out a powerful rep in the gym or jumping, and the lactic acid cycle, which provides energy for longer bouts of high intensity exercise (for up to 3 minutes), such as climbing a steep hill, running a lap of an oval as fast as you can, or doing sit-ups for a full minute. If you've ever felt a 'burn' in your muscles towards the end of an intense exercise, yelling out to you, 'I can't keep this up for much longer!' you're experiencing the by-product of the lactic acid system, called 'lactic acid' — aka: the 'burn' (you'll know it when you feel it!). Bring it on!

7. Set new personal bests — increase intensity

It's important not to stay at the same intensity or on the same program for too long, as your results will plateau.

Once a routine or exercise gets easier, you need to increase the intensity — go faster, have less rest, increase the duration, choose a more challenging exercise, lift a heavier weight — to keep getting continued results. Set small, measurable, achievable training goals on a regular basis. If you ran for 3 minutes last week, aim for 4 minutes the following week. If you've been pedalling on the stationary bike on the same level of resistance, increase it by a level or try an in-built interval program. If you couldn't lift that heavier weight, keep trying until you can! If you've only been able to complete half of that exercise class, next time go for the full class.

The fitter you get, the more you'll be able to push yourself, and you'll need to because your heart rate won't be as high from doing the same workout — a good sign that your cardiovascular system is making adaptations and you're getting fitter!

8. Results come from commitment and consistency

The key to results from any training program is consistency. Always finish what you started. And if you miss a workout, be sure to make it up the next day. No excuses!

One of my favourite sayings is: 'Systems don't fail people, people fail systems'. Commit to the program, be disciplined, stick with it and you will get results!

Program guidelines

The Hard'n Up Training Program is a four-phase program consisting of resistance training and cardio, aimed at fat loss, strength, muscle shape and tone, and overall good health and vitality.

The program will see you through 24 weeks (almost half the year). When you reach the end of the four phases, you return to the beginning and kick off again from Phase 1, this time trying to increase the intensity, level and weight you did before. To follow the program you simply choose from any of the cardio options, and combine it with the four-phase resistance component.

About the cardio component

The type of cardio activity you choose to do will depend on your preference, what cardio equipment you have access to, if you like to do aerobics classes, and what environment you like to do your cardio in — indoors or outdoors.

Train, don't complain!

Phases 1 and 2:

Complete three cardio sessions per week.

Phases 3 and 4:

Complete two to four cardio sessions per week.

Aim: Maximise calorie expenditure for time spent while building cardiovascular health and fitness.

Level: Suitable for all fitness levels.

Program structure: Simply choose from one of the 14 cardio options (see pages 178–181) and complete. Aim to do at least two different options within each week.

About the resistance component

The resistance program requires gym equipment. A gym has all the tools you need to train efficiently as well as access to personal trainers or gym instructors to motivate and support you, and supervise your technique. If your gym doesn't have the equipment prescribed in the exercise, simply replace with a similar exercise that works the same body part.

Phase 1: Weight training

Aim: High-intensity total body workout. Designed for maximum fat loss and muscle tone, using resistance machines.

Level: Suitable for absolute beginners through to advanced exercisers. Beginners should always have a trainer supervising them until they have perfected exercise technique.

Program structure: Total body workout to be done twice per week. Have at least 48 hours' rest between workouts.

Phase 2: Free weight transition

Aim: To provide a smooth transition from machine-based training to free weight lifting. Build body awareness and coordination. Elevate body metabolism and fat burning due to large volume of muscles recruited.

Level: Suitable for intermediate lifters (those that have been training for 3 plus months) or beginners who have completed Phase 1 and can be supervised by a trainer.

'Be the role mode
wanted to be: sto
victim to life, lea
set a good examp
and others — an

you always

playing the

n how to say no,

e for your kids

cut the excuses!'

———————————————————————

Shannan Ponton

Program structure: Total body workouts to be done two to three times per week. Have at least 48 hours' rest between workouts.

Phase 3: Peripheral heart action

Aim: To increase metabolism and cardiac load by working muscles in a specific order — upper body, lower body, then abs. This order ensures your heart has to work extra hard to shunt blood from the upper body, to the lower body and, finally, the abs. This is an excellent training method for fat burning and increasing the load placed on your cardiac system.

Level: Suitable for advanced lifters or those who have completed Phases 1 and 2.

Program structure: Total body workout to be done two to three times per week. Have at least 48 hours' rest between workouts.

Phase 4: Super sets

Aim: Super setting is great for toning and 'cutting up' muscles. This time we're super setting (no rest period) the same muscle group. This allows you to target a specific area and take it much closer to total fatigue. Prepare to burn!

Level: Suitable for advanced lifters or those who have completed Phases 2 and 3.

Program structure: Program 1: Upper Body; Program 2: Lower Body/Abs.

Alternate between these two programs, doing four sessions per week. Can be done on consecutive days; have 48 hours' rest before working the same body part.

Intensity guide — for cardio workouts

To make sure you are working out at a hard enough intensity to reap results, you'll need to measure your exercise intensity. There are two simple ways to monitor your level of exertion.

1. The puff test

How much you puff is a fuss-free indicator of how hard you're working: the harder you puff, the harder you're working and the more calories you're burning. For the bulk of your sessions you should be puffing while still being able to just carry on a conversation. Within this level of intensity you will have moments of training where you're really huffing and puffing and will find it very hard to carry on a conversation.

So long as you're healthy and have a trainer to supervise, don't be afraid to push yourself to this limit.

2. The heart rate test

Measuring your heart rate is a more specific way to measure intensity than relying on your breathing rate. Monitoring how many times your heart beats offers feedback on just how hard you're really working, in other words, you may not be working as hard as you perceive you are! You can measure your heart rate using a clock with a seconds hand or a stopwatch (see page 54 in Part 1), or a heart-rate monitor.

A quick, general intensity guide

Beginners: Make sure you're puffing or have a heart rate at or above 130 bpm (beats per minute).

Intermediate/ advanced: Make sure you're puffing, or have a heart rate at or above 150 bpm, with periods in your training where you're really huffing and puffing.

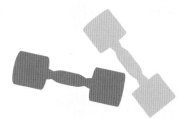

Gear up

If you're after the ultimate training tool, look no further than a heart-rate monitor (two transmitters on a thin strap worn around your chest area close to your heart that talks to a wrist watch). As you exercise, you simply glance at your watch to get an instant heart-rate reading. Heart rate monitors also have other features such as how many calories you burned in a workout. I recommend getting one with heart rate, calorie expenditure and a stopwatch as a minimum. If you can't afford one straight off the bat, why not put it on your Christmas or birthday wish list or make it your reward to yourself for achieving your short-term training and weight-loss goals. But the sooner you get one the better because, like the scales, they're not open to interpretation, emotion or perception. They give you an exact measure of just how hard you are working and how many calories you're burning, so let science do the thinking for you and keep you on track!

For a more specific guide

You can work out your desired percentage of your Maximum Heart Rate (MHR). A heart-rate monitor will do this for you or you can work it out on your own, using the following Karvonen formula.

1. Work out your maximum heart rate (MHR), by subtracting your age from 220: 220 minus age = MHR

For example, if you are 35 years old, your MHR is 220-35 = 185 bpm

2. Next, work out a percentage of your MHR to determine your target heart-rate zone.

For example, if you want to exercise at between 60 and 70 per cent of your MHR, your target heart rate zone is between: (0.6 x 185 = 111 bpm) and (0.7 x 185 = 130 bpm): 111–130 bpm.

While calculating training zones is satisfying to those tech-heads out there and useful as a rough guide for beginners and the average Joe, it can be limiting and hold you back from maximum results. Here's why: an obese person will often get a heart rate in excess of 180 bpm by merely walking to the mail box, which would most likely be close to their maximum heart rate and exceed the recommended heart-rate training zones. Another flaw when using heart-rate zones is the perceived 'fat burning zone' — for years, people believed there was a magical heart-rate range at a low intensity that if you stayed in you knew you were burning fat. This is flawed because although the body burns fat preferentially at low intensities, the best way to achieve fat loss is to burn as many calories as you can, which requires you to get your heart rate up high (not stay within some set zone).

Always remember the golden rule of exercise for weight loss: the harder and faster you go, the higher your heart rate; the higher your heart rate the more calories you burn; the more calories you burn the smaller your butt and tummy will be!

Warm ups and cool downs

I still believe in a good warm-up and cool-down stretch. Debate has raged over the past couple of years as to the validity and timing of stretching. But look at it this way: it never harmed anybody! I believe warming up is essential to prevent injuries and prepare your mind and body before activity. Cooling down helps to lengthen your muscles and help ease muscle stiffness post-workout.

Warming up before a workout involves light intensity activity such as a light jog around the oval, a pedal on the stationary bike, or a couple of easy warm-up sets on a light weight before a weight-training workout. Basic stretches can also be done as part of your warm up, but can be reserved for the end if you prefer. A warm up usually lasts between around 5–10 minutes and is essential for:

• Gradually increasing your heart rate.

• Pumping oxygenated blood to the required working muscles.

• Preparing your body for the workout ahead.

• Limbering muscles and joints.

• Reducing the risk of injury.

Cooling down involves around 5 minutes of light intensity activity such as a gentle jog or walk, or gradually winding down the intensity of your workout in stages, followed by a series of stretches. Depending on the length of the stretch component, a cool down will usually last 10–15 minutes. This wind-down period is essential for:

• Returning your heart, breathing and blood pressure to pre-exercise levels.

• Preventing dizziness.

• Ridding waste products such as lactic acid from your muscles.

• Improving flexibility.

• Helping you back up for tomorrow's workout with less stiffness and pain.

• Reducing the risk of injury.

Resistance rules — for resistance workouts

Here are some tips and guidelines for general weight training and following the four-phase resistance program.

1. Be sure to read through the exercise descriptions in the next chapter. If you're still unsure how to do an exercise or are new to weight training, have a personal trainer, gym instructor or experienced training partner teach you correct technique, and watch you until you are competent and confident with each exercise.

2. Never sacrifice technique for weight. Meaning: never choose a weight that is too heavy to allow you to perform the exercise with perfect technique. This not only defeats the purpose by possibly bringing other muscles into play — for example, arching your back to give an extra 'oomph' to a bicep curl — but puts you at risk of incurring an injury.

3. Write down each and every set that you perform (space is provided on the resistance program), including what weight you lifted and for how many repetitions. This makes it much easier for you to remember the appropriate weight for the next session, and to see your increases in black and white — it's very motivating to look back and see how much stronger you're getting!

4. If you feel that your form is not perfect or you think that an injury may be developing, ask for advice immediately. Don't keep doing an exercise if it feels wrong or uncomfortable. Get it sorted out.

5. Quality matters more than quantity when it comes to weight training. You don't need to be in the gym for hours on end. Each of the workouts should take only 40–50 minutes.

6. Never hold your breath when you're lifting weights. This can cause a dangerous rise in blood pressure and should be avoided. As a general rule, breathe out on the grunt (exertion) phase and breath in as you return to the start position of the exercise or in between each rep. The most important thing is to keep breathing!

7. Concentration is essential when lifting weights. It's not a time for chit-chat. Think about the muscle you're targeting, mentally focus on the muscle, and feel its movement as you perform each repetition. This is called the mind muscle connection, and helps you pinpoint the target muscles and work them more effectively.

8. Get a 'spot'. Having someone 'spot' you not only ensures safe technique, it helps you push out that extra repetition you wouldn't have been able to on your own — helping you make further strength gains.

9. When doing abdominal exercises, always contract your stomach (pull your belly button inwards towards your spine) and hold this contraction through the entire movement.

10. Brace your core and maintain the natural curve of your spine. Whether you're standing, sitting or lying when lifting, always keep your deep stomach muscles 'turned on' and engaged — this helps set up the correct curvature of the spine, prevent injury and get more from your lift.

Trainer talk

To help you navigate your way around the training programs and increase your understanding of important training terms here's a list of trainer's lingo explained.

Compound exercise:

A big muscle exercise. Any exercise requiring you to move more than one muscle group and joint is called a compound exercise. For example, when you do a push-up you're moving two joints (elbow and shoulder joints) and working more than one muscle group: arms, chest (pectorals) and shoulders.

Isolated exercise:

A single muscle exercise. Any exercise involving one muscle group and joint movement. For example, when you do a bicep curl you're moving one joint (elbow joint) and working one muscle group (biceps).

Super set:

Doing two or more exercises in a row, followed by a rest break. These exercises may work the same muscle group or opposing muscle groups.

Progressive overload:

Gradually increasing the intensity or load of an exercise/program in a step-like fashion so your body progresses through three stages: overload, adaptation, and improvement.

Reps:

Short for repetitions — how many times you do an exercise. For example: 'Drop and give me 20 push-ups!' translates to 20 reps of push-ups.

Sets:

The amount of times you complete a set of reps. For example: 'Now give me another 20 push-ups' translates to two sets of 20 reps.

Failure:

Pushing your muscles to a point of failure whereby you literally cannot do another rep of the exercise.

Get a 'spot':

A spotter is an experienced training partner or personal trainer who supervises a heavy/hard exercise by watching your technique and giving a little assistance to push out that last rep.

Prone position:

Lying face down.

Supine position:

Lying face up (on your back).

Pronated grip:

Overhand grip.

Supinated grip:

Underhand grip.

Split routine:

Dividing your weight-training program into body parts or sections over a set training period. For example, a split routine of upper body and lower body exercises, or a split program of chest and tris; back and bis; shoulders, abs and legs.

Plyometrics:

Stretching a muscle before firing it such as bending down into a semi-squat and then jumping up high. Think explosive power movements.

EZ bar:

Also EZ curl bar or E Z bar, a variation of a barbell with a curve in the bar where you grip it. It's designed to take the strain off your wrists.

Incline bench:

A bench seat used for lifting weights, which reclines back to a set angle — usually 30 degrees.

Fartlek:

A Swedish term meaning 'speed play'. A loosely structured form of interval training involving a continuous cardio session with bursts of strenuous, high intensity periods such as going for a run and doing random sprint bursts throughout.

Muscle hypertrophy:

An increase in muscle size as a result of an increase in the size of your muscle fibres, rather than an increase in the number of muscle fibres (hyperplasia).

DOMS:

Stands for 'Delayed Onset of Muscle Soreness' — the pain you feel in your muscles after a hard training session, usually 24–48 hours later. In other words, that face-grimacing feeling of trying to get up off your chair or walk down a set of stairs after a tough leg workout!

Cross-training:

Training in different ways, which vary to your usual exercise program. For example, doing boxing as a form of cross-training if you're on a running program. This gives the muscles that you typically use in your standard workout a break, while still maintaining conditioning. Cross-training can also refer to doing different exercises that focus on different body parts within the same workout, for example, a cross-training cardio circuit in the gym of 20 minutes on the treadmill, 20 minutes on the rower, and 20 minutes on the stationary bike.

Cardio plus Weights plus Recovery equals guaranteed weight loss and an awesome body

If you just train, train, train, with no recovery and relaxation, your body may suffer in the way of an injury or burn out. Take time out of your training to replenish, rejuvenate, and allow your muscles to recover and make adaptations from your effort. Some great ways to do this include stretching, yoga, massage, swimming, meditatation, cross-training for active recovery or surfing (my personal favourite!).

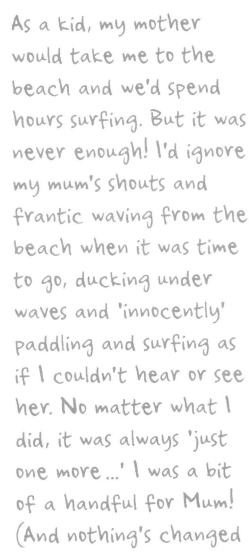

As a kid, my mother would take me to the beach and we'd spend hours surfing. But it was never enough! I'd ignore my mum's shouts and frantic waving from the beach when it was time to go, ducking under waves and 'innocently' paddling and surfing as if I couldn't hear or see her. No matter what I did, it was always 'just one more...' I was a bit of a handful for Mum! (And nothing's changed ... there's always room for 'just one more ...')

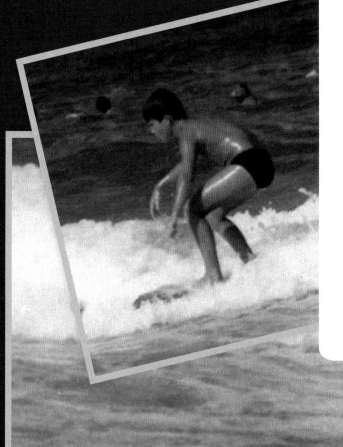

Chapter 9:
Build UP —
The Hard'n Up
Toolbox

Now you know more about the plan, you need the programs, nuts and bolts (exercises and stretches) to execute the plan and build your new body. Here you'll find everything you need to put the Hard'n Up Training Program together: the training programs, cardio exercises, resistance exercises and stretches.

Remember to ease into your program and progress the intensity gradually. It's no use getting so sore that you can't finish the full week's program.

The training programs

Combine any of the 14 options in the cardio program (pages 178–181) with the four-phase resistance program (pages 188). Follow the instruction guidelines to follow for each of the four phases in The Hard'n Up Training Program. You can find the exercises and stretches you need for the training programs after the programs on pages 192–221.

Space has been provided for you to record your workout results on the resistance programs. If you want to log your cardio workout results, simply log them in a training diary or use the Cardio Log in Part 4, Chapter 12, 'Tools to keep you on track — Diaries, logs and planners'.

Phase 1: Hard'n Up Training Program

Cardio

- What? Choose from any of the cardio options.

- How many times per week? 3. (Do at least 2 different cardio workouts within the week.)

- Instruction: Follow the instructions as outlined in your chosen cardio option.

- Progression: Aim to improve your intensity, level and/ or speed each week by following the suggested progression for your chosen cardio option.

Resistance

- What? Complete the Phase 1: Weight training program (page 182).

- How many times per week? 2. Have at least 48 hours' rest in between resistance workouts.

- Rest periods:
1 minute between each group of exercises; 30 seconds rest only between each set. For example, for machine chest press, do 12 reps, rest 30 seconds; 10 reps, rest 30 seconds; 8 reps, rest 30 seconds; 6 reps, rest 30 seconds, then rest for 1 minute and move on to lat pull down. NOTE: The last exercise group is done as a super set, so do 12 reps standing tricep pushdown, followed (no rest) by 12 reps dumbbell bicep curl, rest 30 seconds, do 10 reps standing tricep pushdown and dumbbell bicep curl (no rest in between), rest 30 seconds, do 8 reps and so on.

- Progression:
Week 1–2: Perform 12, 10, 8, 6 repetitions. Choose a weight so that you can just finish each set. The weight should increase slightly for each set.

Week 3–6: Perform 12, 10, 8, 6 repetitions. Choose a weight so that you can just finish each set. Rest for 30 seconds and return the weight to your 8 or 10 repetition weight, then do one gut-busting set to absolute failure! (Approximately 12–15 repetitions.)

Phase 2: Hard'n Up Training Program

Cardio

- What? Choose from any of the cardio options.

- How many times per week? 3. (Do at least 2 different cardio workouts in the week.)

- Instruction: Follow the instructions as outlined in your chosen cardio option.

- Progression: Aim to improve your intensity, level and/or speed each week by following the suggested progression for your chosen cardio option.

Resistance

- What? Complete the Phase 2: Free Weight Transition program (page 184).

- How many times per week? 2-3 sessions. Have at least 48 hours' rest in between resistance workouts.

- Rest periods:
1 minute between sets and exercises. (Abdominal exercises to be done in between this one minute rest period where indicated in the program.) For example, do 1 set of 10 reps bench press, do 10 repetitions of the specified ab exercise, 1 set of 10 reps bench press, 10 reps of abs, 1 set of 10 reps bench press, 10 reps of abs, rest 1 minute then move on to barbell squats.

- Progression:
Choose a weight such that you can successfully complete 3 sets of 10 repetitions. Once you can complete 3 sets of 10 repetitions, increase the weight slightly. When you first increase the weight, you may not be able to get 3 sets of 10 out (for example, you might only be able to do 10, 9, 8 repetitions), but do as many as you can and stay at this weight until you can once again complete the full 3 sets of 10. Then increase the weight again and repeat the process.

Phase 3: Hard'n Up Training Program

Cardio

- What? Choose from any of the cardio options.

- How many times per week? 2–4. (Do at least 2 different cardio workouts in the week).

- Instruction: Follow the instructions as outlined in your chosen cardio option.

- Progression: Aim to improve your intensity, level and/or speed each week by following the suggested progression for your chosen cardio option.

Resistance

- What? Complete the Phase 3: Peripheral Heart Action program.

- How many times per week? 2–3. Have at least 48 hours' rest in between resistance workouts.

- Rest periods:
Each group of exercises are done as super sets, which means you work upper body, lower body then abs with no rest in between each exercise. Once you have completed this pattern, rest for 1 minute before repeating another set of exercises as a super set. Each group is to be completed three times before moving onto the next group, taking a 1-minute rest between each group. For example, in weeks 1 and 2 you do 3 sets of 10 reps for all exercises. You would do 10 reps flat dumbbell chest press, followed by 10 reps dumbbell squats, followed by 10 reps bosu crunch with no rest in between. Rest for 1 minute and repeat this super set again, rest for 1 minute and repeat again. Rest for one minute then move on to the next super set of seated row, lying leg curl, V-sit and follow the same pattern.

- Progression:
  Week 1-2: Choose a weight that you can just complete 3 sets of 10 repetitions with.

  Week 3-4: Keep the same weight but now complete 3 sets of 12 repetitions.

  Week 5-6: Maintain the same weight as the previous 4 weeks, for 3 sets of 15 repetitions. This program increases the intensity of your workout by increasing the number of repetitions. By weeks 5 and 6 you are lifting 50 per cent more than your starting weight. It's hard work but definitely achievable — and worth it in the end!

Phase 4: Hard'n Up Training Program

Cardio

- What? Choose from any of the cardio options.

- How many times per week? 2-4. (Do at least 2 different cardio workouts in the week).

- Instruction: Follow the instructions as outlined in your chosen cardio option.

- Progression: Aim to improve your intensity, level and/or speed each week by following the suggested progression for your chosen cardio option.

Resistance

- What? Complete the Phase 4: Super sets program (page 188).

- How many times per week? 4 in total — alternate between program 1 (upper body) and program 2 (lower body/abs). Can be done on consecutive days but have at least 48 hours' rest in between the same body part (program).

- Rest periods: Muscle groups are done as super sets (no rest). Rest 1 minute between super sets and 1 minute between body parts. For example, do 12 reps incline dumbbell chest press followed by 12 reps incline dumbbell flyes, rest 1 minute then repeat 12 reps incline dumbbell chest press followed by 12 reps

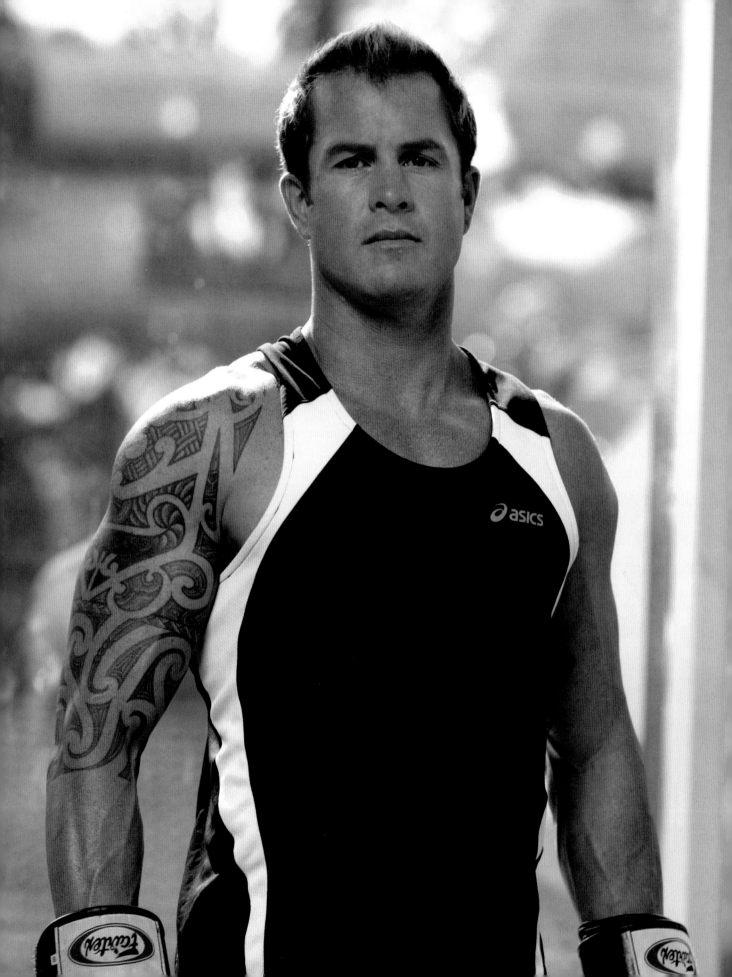

incline dumbbell flyes, rest
1 minute then repeat one more
time. Rest one minute then start
next body part.

- Progression:
Weeks 1–2: Start with a weight
(body weight for ab exercises)
that you can just complete 3 sets
of 12 repetitions with.

Week 3: Increase your weight
slightly and complete 3 sets of
12 repetitions.

Week 4: Maintain the same weight
as the previous week and try to
complete 3 sets of 15 repetitions.

Weeks 5–6: If you managed to
squeeze out 3 sets of 15 in week
4 increase your weight slightly,
if not work towards finishing 3 sets
of 15 repetitions before increasing
your weight slightly. By weeks 5
and 6 you should be taking your
muscles to complete failure.

How to fill in the resistance program charts

Follow the guidelines on sets, rest periods and reps for the week you're at in each of the 4 phases. The amount of reps and sets you need to do is repeated again in the chart as a quick reminder. Photocopy the charts and take the program to the gym; by keeping a blank template in the book you can make as many copies as you like and re-use the chart if you repeat any of the phases. Space has been provided for you to record your workout results, simply fill in the reps you completed in one half of the set box and the weight you lifted in the other half (for example, in Phase 1, if you did 12 reps on your first set of machine chest press at 15 kilograms, you write 12/15 in the Set 1 box; where you use your body weight, such as sit-ups, just record the reps or write BW for body weight). This will highlight the improvements you make over the weeks as well as give you a quick cue as to what weight to use on your next workout. In Phase 1, weeks 1–2, you won't use all of the five set boxes as you're only required to do 4 sets in total so leave the Set 5 boxes blank, then use the Set 5 boxes in Weeks 3–6 when you're required to do 5 sets in total.

Cardio program

Type:	Treadmill intervals
Instruction:	Run 30 seconds, rest 30 seconds (standing feet astride the moving belt). Gradually build your speed until you reach your peak. Continue performing 30 run: 30 rest second intervals for 20 plus minutes.
Progression:	Each time you repeat the workout try to increase your top speed.
Type:	Rowing
Instruction:	Row 500 metres as fast as you can. This becomes your benchmark time. Rest 1 minute and try to 'beat' your first time. Repeat this 6 times (Ouch!).
Progression:	Aim to increase your personal best benchmark time.
Type:	Treadmill/Cross-trainer
Instruction:	Start at a comfortable level, every minute increase your speed for 5 minutes. By the time you reach 5 minutes, you should be at your max physically and/or your heart rate should be up. Without any rest, decrease the speed on the minute for the next 5 minutes. Rest 2 minutes then repeat.
Progression:	Aim to increase the speed you can reach at 5 minutes.
Type:	Start moving at a medium-fast pace. Every minute on the minute for 10 minutes increase the incline/resistance, aiming to maintain the same speed. At 10 minutes, go as fast and hard as you can for one more 1 minute interval. Rest 1 minute and work your way back down the incline/resistance each minute on the minute until you reach 0.
Progression:	Aim to increase the incline/resistance.

Cardio program

Type:	Rowing
Instruction:	Row for maximum distance in 2 minutes. Rest for 1 minute. In the initial rest period perform 1 push-up, 1 crunch, 1 squat jump. Start second 2 minute rowing interval, try to match your first distance, then perform 2 push-ups, 2 crunches, 2 squat jumps within the 1 minute rest. Third interval of 2 minutes, 3 of each, etc.
Progression:	Aim to get to 10 intervals. Now there's a challenge for the elite!

Type:	Hills
Instruction:	Find a long, fairly steep hill. Walk, run or cycle up, return to the bottom at a steady pace, and repeat for 20 minutes.
Progression:	Increase the amount of hills you're able to complete in 20 minutes. Advanced exercisers: Aim to keep your heart rate above 170 bpm in the work interval.

Type:	Stair session
Instruction:	Find a set of stairs in your apartment building, office, at the local park or footy field or even at home. • Run or walk up the stairs, one step at a time, then return to the bottom. • Run or walk up the stairs, two steps at a time, then return to the bottom. • Run or walk up the stairs, three steps at a time (providing they're not too far apart), then return to the bottom. • Repeat the entire sequence for 20 minutes.
Progression:	Increase the amount of flights you're able to complete in 20 minutes. Advanced exercisers: Aim to keep your heart rate above 170 bpm in the work interval.

Cardio program

Type:	Exercise class
Instruction:	Choose from: Body Attack, Spin, Basic Training, Body Combat, Boot Camp, Hi-NRG Aerobic, Circuit, Boxing Class
Progression:	Aim to complete a full class; push yourself harder each class; take on a more challenging class.

Type:	Team or individual sport
Instruction:	Training session; competition or game.
Progression:	

Type:	Fast power walk
Instruction:	Walk for 60 minutes, keeping heart rate above 120 bpm.
Progression:	Vary your path to include hills or walk for longer.

Type:	Jog
Instruction:	Jog for 30 minutes, keeping heart rate above 160 bpm.
Progression:	Vary your running route to include hills.

Type:	Jog
Instruction:	40 minute jog/walk, keeping heart rate above 140 bpm.
Progression:	Bridge the gap between walking and running so you run more than you walk

Cardio program

Type:	Cardio triathlon
Instruction:	10 minute treadmill, 10 minute rower, 10 minute cross-trainer, keeping heart rate above 160 bpm.
Progression:	Aim to increase distance covered, speed, duration, heart rate and calorie expenditure.

Type:	Boxing pyramid done on a heavy bag or focus pads with a partner.
Instruction:	• 10 punches, 1 push-up, then 20 punches, 2 push-ups, continue this pattern up to 100 punches, 10 push-ups. Change partners. • Next: 50 punches, run 10 metres, 20 punching sit-ups (partner holds focus pads above your knees as you sit up punch left, right then down and repeat), run back and repeat for 2 minutes, then change over so your partner completes the same 2 minute interval. Next, substitute sit-ups with squat jumps, tricep dips and finally burpees.
Progression:	Work your way up to completing the entire workout, for at least 40 minutes.

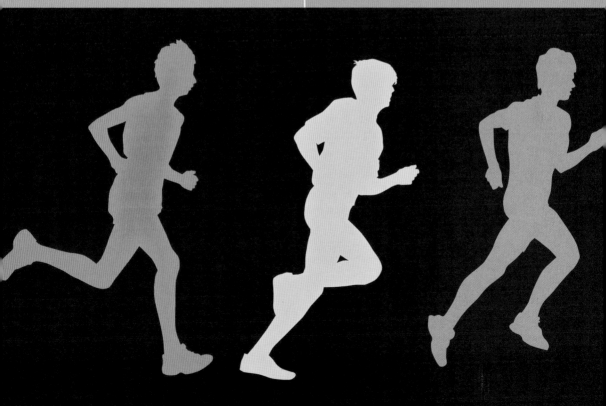

PHASE 1: Resistance program

Phase 1: Weight Training Body part: Total Body	Date	Set 1	Set 2	Set 3	Set 4	Set 5	Set 1	Set 2	Set 3	Set 4	Set 5	Set 1	Set 2	Set 3	Set 4	Set 5	Set 1	Set 2	Set 3	Set 4	Set 5
Machine chest press																					
Lat pull down																					
Machine shoulder press																					
Smith machine squats																					

Lying leg curl

Set 1												
Set 2												
Set 3												
Set 4												
Set 5												

Standing tricep pushdown

Set 1												
Set 2												
Set 3												
Set 4												
Set 5												

super set with

Dumbbell bicep curl

Set 1												
Set 2												
Set 3												
Set 4												
Set 5												

Instruction:

- Rest 30 seconds in between sets and 1 minute in between each set group
- Weeks 1-2: 12, 10, 8, 6 reps (4 sets in total)
- Weeks 3-6: 12, 10, 8, 6, plus 1 set to failure (aim for 12-15 reps using your 8-10 rep weight) (5 sets in total)

PHASE 2: Resistance program

Phase 2: Free Weight
Transition
Body part: Total Body

Date	Set 1	Set 2	Set 3		Set 1	Set 2	Set 3	Set 1	Set 2	Set 3		Set 1	Set 2	Set 3	Set 1	Set 2	Set 3	Set 1	Set 2	Set 3
Flat bench press				**+**	**Crunch**			**Barbell squats**			**+**	**Oblique crunch**			**Chin-ups/Assisted Chin-ups**			**Romanian dead lift**		

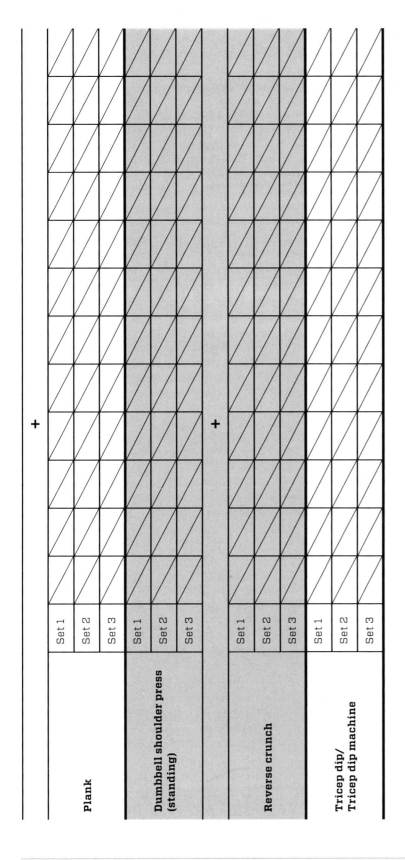

		Set 1																
Plank		Set 2																
		Set 3																
Dumbbell shoulder press (standing)		Set 1																
		Set 2																
		Set 3																
Reverse crunch		Set 1																
		Set 2																
		Set 3																
Tricep dip/ Tricep dip machine		Set 1																
		Set 2																
		Set 3																

Instruction:

- Rest 1 minute in between sets and exercises (do ab exercises within this rest period)
- Do 3 sets of 10 reps for each weight-training exercise and ab exercise (except for plank: do 3 sets of 30 second holds)
- Increase the weight used for each weight-training exercise once you can do 3 sets of 10 reps

PHASE 3: Resistance program

Phase 3: Peripheral Heart Action Body part: Total Body	Date												
Flat dumbbell chest press	Set 1												
	Set 2												
	Set 3												
super set with													
Dumbbell squats	Set 1												
	Set 2												
	Set 3												
super set with													
Bosu crunch	Set 1												
	Set 2												
	Set 3												
Seated row	Set 1												
	Set 2												
	Set 3												
super set with													
Lying leg curl	Set 1												
	Set 2												
	Set 3												
super set with													
V-sit	Set 1												
	Set 2												
	Set 3												
Swiss ball dumbbell press	Set 1												
	Set 2												
	Set 3												
super set with													
Walking dumbbell lunges	Set 1												
	Set 2												
	Set 3												

		super set with														
Swiss ball crunch	Set 1															
	Set 2															
	Set 3															
Seated dumbbell extension	Set 1															
	Set 2															
	Set 3															

		super set with														
Dumbbell step-ups	Set 1															
	Set 2															
	Set 3															

		super set with														
Incline reverse crunch	Set 1															
	Set 2															
	Set 3															
Standing E-Z bar curl	Set 1															
	Set 2															
	Set 3															

		super set with														
Lying E-Z bar extension	Set 1															
	Set 2															
	Set 3															

		super set with														
Bicycle crunch	Set 1															
	Set 2															
	Set 3															

Instruction:

- Do all three exercises as a super set with no rest in between, rest for one minute; repeat this sequence twice before moving on to the next super set group
- Weeks 1-2: Do 3 sets of 10 reps
- Weeks 3-4: Do 3 sets of 12 reps
- Weeks 5-6: Do 3 sets of 15 reps

PHASE 4: Resistance program 1

Phase 4: Super Sets
Body part: Upper body

Date										

Incline dumbbell chest press	Set 1									
	Set 2									
	Set 3									

super set with

Incline dumbbell flyes	Set 1									
	Set 2									
	Set 3									

Straight arm pull down	Set 1									
	Set 2									
	Set 3									

super set with

Lat pull down	Set 1									
	Set 2									
	Set 3									

Dumbbell shoulder press (seated)	Set 1									
	Set 2									
	Set 3									

super set with

Exercise		Set 1	Set 2	Set 3											
Dumbbell side raises		Set 1	Set 2	Set 3											
Tricep dip		Set 1	Set 2	Set 3											

super set with

Exercise		Set 1	Set 2	Set 3											
Standing rope pullover		Set 1	Set 2	Set 3											
Standing E-Z bar curl		Set 1	Set 2	Set 3											

super set with

Exercise		Set 1	Set 2	Set 3											
Hammer curl		Set 1	Set 2	Set 3											

Instruction:

- Exercises done together as a super set. Rest 1 minute between super sets and body parts
- Weeks 1-3: 3 sets of 12 reps
- Week 4-6: 3 sets of 15 reps

BUILD UP — THE HARD'N UP TOOLBOX

PHASE 4: Resistance program 2

Phase 4: Super Sets
Body part: Lower body/Abs

Date			
Leg press	Set 1	Set 2	Set 3
super set with			
Leg extension	Set 1	Set 2	Set 3
Smith machine lunges	Set 1	Set 2	Set 3
super set with			
Dumbbell dead lift	Set 1	Set 2	Set 3
Lying leg curl	Set 1	Set 2	Set 3
super set with			

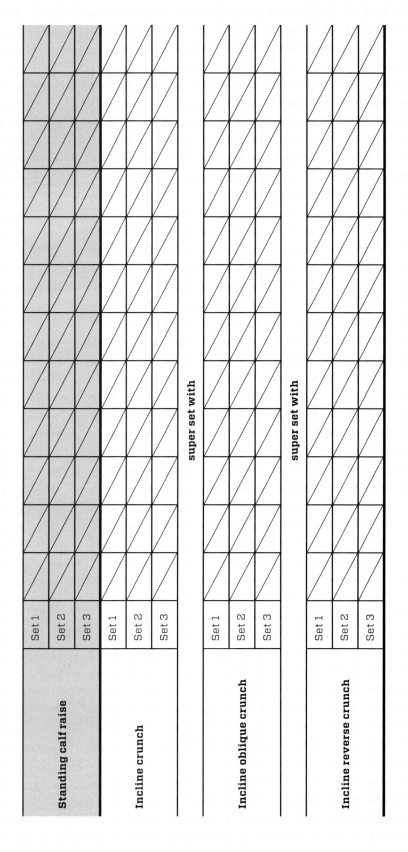

Standing calf raise	Set 1											
	Set 2											
	Set 3											

super set with

Incline crunch	Set 1											
	Set 2											
	Set 3											

Incline oblique crunch	Set 1											
	Set 2											
	Set 3											

super set with

Incline reverse crunch	Set 1											
	Set 2											
	Set 3											

Instruction:

- Exercises done together as a super set.
- Rest 1 minute between super sets and body parts
- Weeks 1-3: 3 sets of 12 reps
- Week 4-6: 3 sets of 15 reps

The exercises

Body part: Chest

The main chest muscles are known as the pectoralis — or the pecs. They consist of the pectoralis major (pec major), which covers the whole chest, and the pectoralis minor (pec minor) which is a smaller muscle lying underneath the pec major.

Dumbbell flyes

Lie on your back on a bench, brace your core and maintain the natural curvature of your spine. Hold both dumbbells facing each other above your chest, with a slight bend in your arms. Take dumbbells out to the sides of your chest, until your chest is slightly stretched. Bring dumbbells back together in a hugging action and repeat.

Technique tip: Be careful not to hyperextend (extend your joint beyond its normal range) the shoulder joint.

Variation: Incline dumbbell flyes

Complete dumbbell flyes lying back on an incline bench — set at about a 30-degree angle.

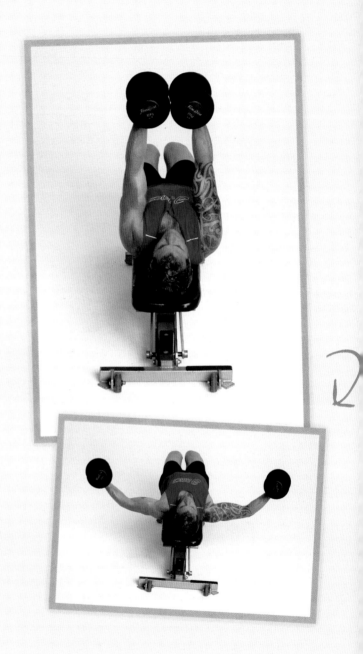

Flat bench press

Lie with your back on a flat bench so the bar sits above your nipple line. Beginners or those with lower back problems, position feet flat on the bench; advanced lifters, position feet on the floor. Grip the bar in a pronated grip with hands slightly wider than shoulder width. Brace your stomach and move the bar off the rack. Position the bar over your chest, arms fully extended. Lower the bar to your chest in a slow and controlled manner, keeping the wrists straight. Pause with the bar a fist width off your chest, then push the bar back up to the start position. Repeat.

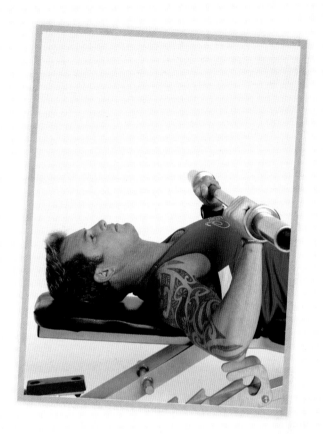

Technique tip: Do not arch your lower back or push your back into the bench (maintain the natural curvature of your spine); do not let your elbows bend past 90 degrees.

Variations: Dumbbell chest press

Hold dumbbells on your chest with palms facing forwards and complete the same action as above. Do on a flat bench (flat dumbbell chest press) on an incline bench set at about a 30-degree angle (incline dumbbell chest press).

Machine chest press

Sit in the chair with knees bent and feet flat on the floor. Position hands on the handles. Keep your shoulders back and down and stomach braced. Push the handles until your elbows are almost straight (not locked), slowly return to the start position and repeat.

Technique tip: Avoid bending elbows past 90 degrees.

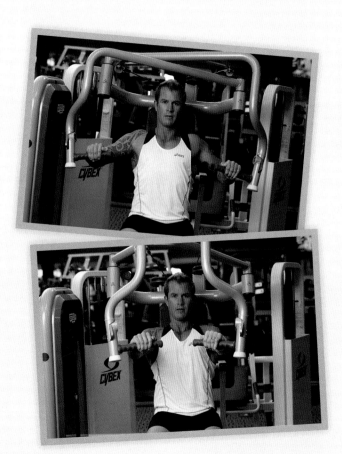

Push-ups

Place hands shoulder width apart, fingers facing forwards, legs out straight behind you and the balls of your feet on the ground. Keep your body in a straight line from head to heel (no sagging stomachs or hunched shoulders). Lower your chest towards the floor by bending your elbows outwards until your chest is a fist width off the ground. Push back up and repeat.

Technique tip: Keep your abs braced. Lower to a shallow depth at first and go deeper as you get stronger.

Variation: Modified push-ups

Even beginners can start on their toes, just limit the depth. You may start only being able to lower a couple of centimetres; as you get stronger go a little deeper. But people with injuries should do modified push-ups — simply place your knees on the ground to make a straight diagonal line from head to knees. Complete the push-up as normal.

Body part: Back

The back muscles consist of the latissimus dorsi — AKA the lats — which can be thought of as the wings that fan out across your back; the rhomboids and trapezius which reside in the upper back; and the erector spinae which runs vertically along the length of your spine, providing support. Strong back muscles are a must for perfect posture.

Assisted chin-ups

Start with assisted chin-ups and work your way up to the real thing. You can either do these on an assisted chin-up machine (place bent knees on the pad and complete a chin-up as usual) or with a trainer supporting your feet to help you up and down.

Chin-ups

Hold a chin-up bar in a closed, pronated grip with hands wider than shoulder width. Lift your feet off the ground, knees bent and feet hooked together. Pull yourself up until your chin reaches the bar, slowly lower your body and repeat.

Technique tip: Maintain correct posture and don't round your upper back. Squeeze your shoulder blades together at the top of the movement to get more from your lift.

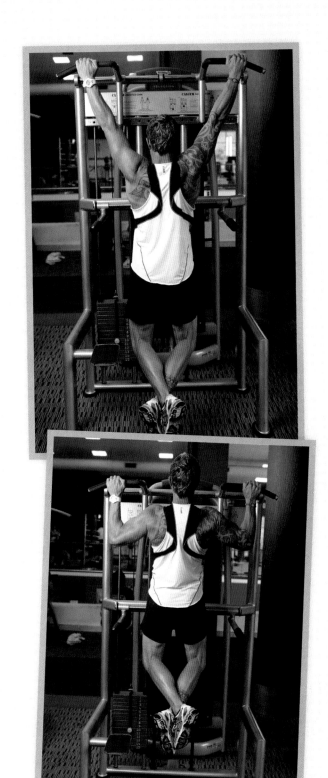

Lat pull down

Stand in front of the lat pull down machine. Hold bar with a closed, pronated, shoulder-width grip. Pull the bar down as you sit down with thighs underneath the pads (or if you have a training partner or trainer, they can pull the bar down for you). Start with your arms fully extended. Pull the bar down to just below your chin, keep a natural curve in your spine with your chest high and 'proud', squeezing your elbows in to your ribs. Slowly raise the bar to start position and repeat.

Technique tip: Keep your chest high and pull the bar down just below your chin.

Seated row

Sit with knees bent, feet placed flat on the foot rests and back upright. Lean forwards and hold the handles in a wide pronated grip, more than shoulder width. Pull your shoulders back and down, holding this position throughout the exercise. Squeeze your shoulder blades together, keeping the natural curve in your spine with your chest high and 'proud' as you pull the handles into your body. Release and return to starting position in a slow and controlled manner and repeat.

Technique tip: Imagine squeezing a walnut in between your shoulder blades as you row back, to get more from the exercise.

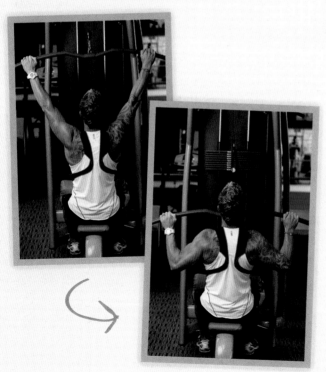

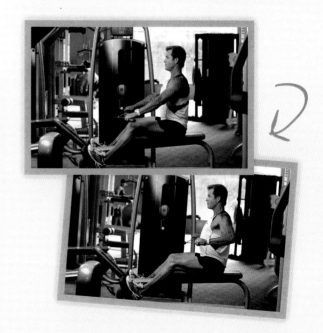

Straight arm pull down

Stand in front of a lat pull down machine
with one foot forwards, one foot back. Hold
the bar with a closed, pronated shoulder-
width grip. Keeping your arms straight,
the natural curve in your spine with
your chest high and 'proud', pull the bar
down towards your thighs, squeeze your
shoulder blades together. Slowly raise the
bar to start position and repeat.

Technique tip: Brace your abs and lean
slightly forwards.

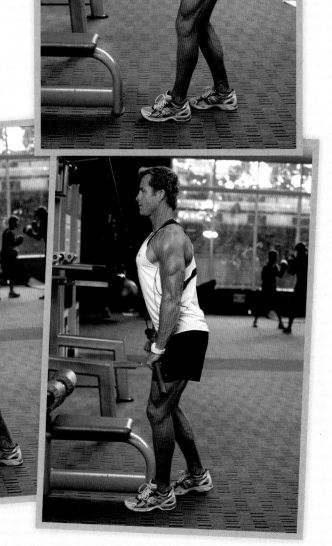

Body part: Arms

Your arms are made up of your biceps or 'bis' (AKA 'guns') which sit on the front of your upper arm and your triceps or 'tris' which sit on the back of your upper arm. Whether you're male or female, toned arms are an essential for summer dressing!

Dumbbell bicep curl

Sit with feet hip-width apart, knees bent. Hold dumbbells by your sides. Curl the dumbbells up to the front of your shoulders, slowly lower and repeat.

Technique tip: Keep your torso upright, abs braced, and focus on using only the bicep muscle to curl the weight up.

Variations: Do a dumbbell bicep curl from a standing position with one foot forward and one foot back.

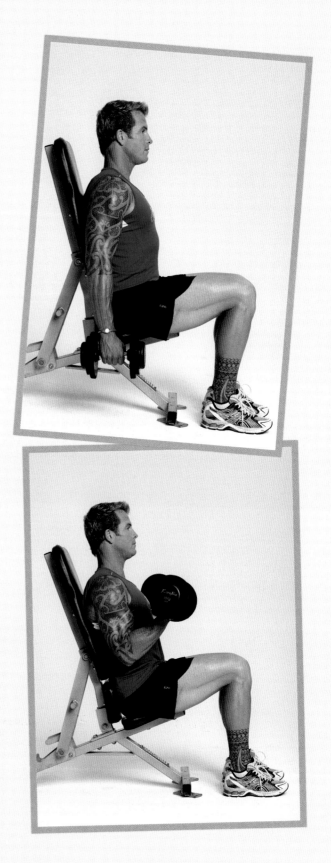

Hammer curl

Complete the same action as a bicep curl with palms facing in and thumbs pointing up.

Technique tip: Lift and lower the dumbbells slowly to avoid momentum and maximise the movement.

Lying E-Z bar extension

Lie on your back on a bench and grab the bar with palms facing forwards. Position the bar above your head, arms straight and running in line with your ears. Keep your elbows fixed and acting like a 'door hinge', lower the bar behind your head by bending your elbows. Straighten your arms and take the bar back up and repeat.

Technique tip: Lower the bar only to your forehead or just past the line of your head.

Variations:

- Use a barbell
- Use two dumbbells, palms facing each other

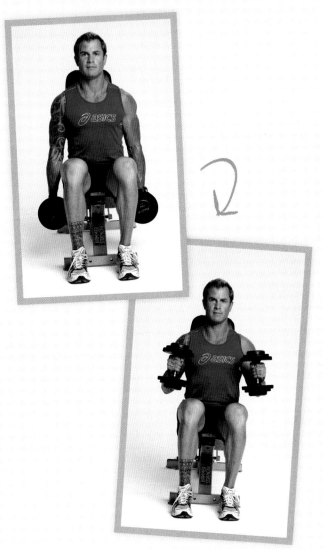

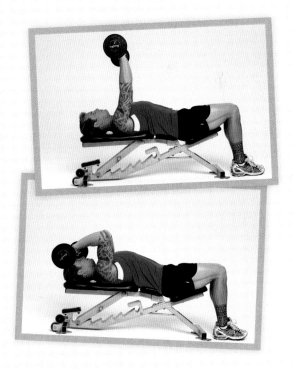

Seated dumbbell extension

Sit upright on an incline bench so it supports your back. Hold one dumbbell with both of your hands positioned just under the top of the weighted part and the shaft of the dumbbell hanging vertically between your thumbs (hands in a 'reverse cup' position). Position the dumbbell straight up over your head with elbows slightly bent. Bend your elbows and lower the dumbbell vertically behind the back of your head until your upper arms go back as far as they can. Squeeze the dumbbell back up to the start position, focusing on using your triceps and repeat.

Technique tip: Always select a weight that will allow you to perform a full range of motion.

Standing E-Z bar curl

Do a bicep curl, holding an E-Z bar. Use a barbell if you don't have access to an E-Z bar.

Technique tip: When doing a standing E-Z bar curl stand with one foot forwards and one foot back to avoid rocking your torso which should stay still throughout the movement.

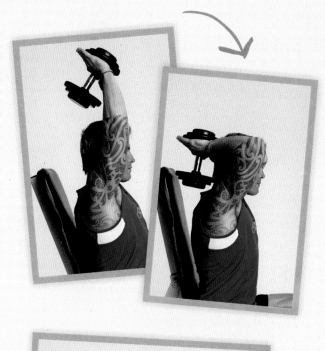

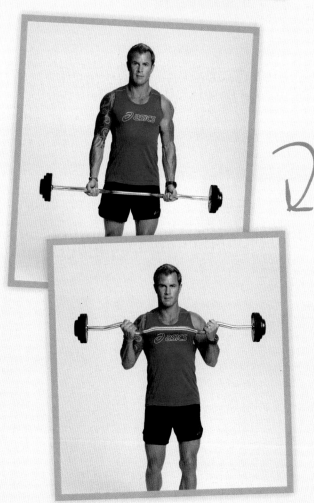

Standing rope pullover

Stand facing away from cable machine with rope placed on the low pulley. Grasp the rope in each hand, stand up tall, elbows bent with the rope just behind your neck. Extend your upper arms until your elbows are fully extended, arms straight and next to your ears. Lower the rope back down behind your neck and repeat.

Technique tip: To avoid pressure in the lower back, lean slightly forwards and brace your abs.

Standing tricep pushdown

Stand in front of the machine with elbows tucked in, one foot forwards, one foot back. Hold handles out in front so elbows are roughly at right angles. Keep elbows tucked in, push the rope (or handles down) until your elbows are straight. Slowly release and repeat.

Technique tip: Your elbow joint is the only joint that should be moving (think door hinge), keep everything else braced.

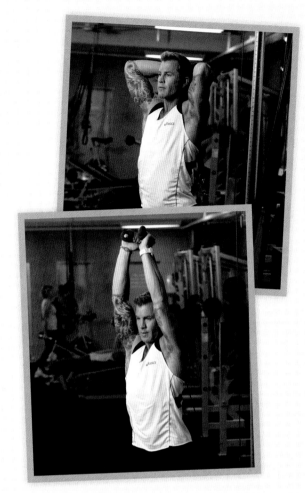

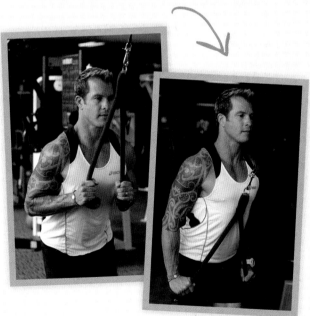

Tricep dip machine

Before attempting tricep dips, start with tricep dip machine.

Sit inside the machine and grasp the handles by the sides of your body. Keep your elbows close to your body, shoulders back and down, back upright, push the handles down until your arms are straight, without locking your elbows, and repeat.

Technique tip: Lower slowly and don't bend elbows past 90 degrees.

Tricep dip

Sit on the edge of a chair or bench, fingers curled over the edge. Slide your backside off, holding your weight through your hands. Bend your elbows (pointing behind), lower. Straighten elbows and push back up and repeat.

Technique tip: Don't use your legs to help you push back up, use the triceps only.

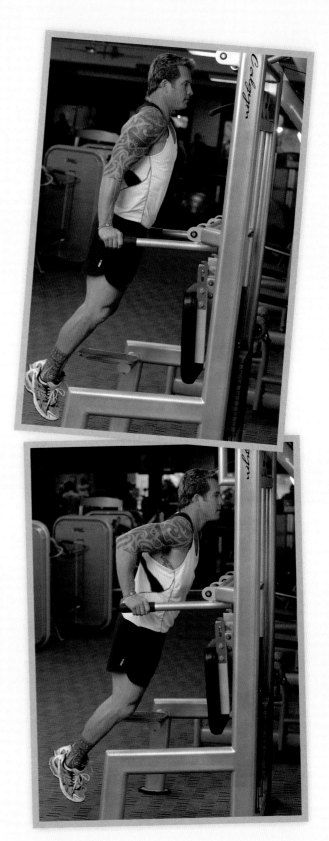

Body part: Shoulders

The shoulders are made up of the deltoids ('delts'): anterior (front deltoid), middle deltoid, and posterior (rear deltoid).

Dumbbell forward raises

Stand with one foot forwards, one foot back and bend knees slightly. Hold dumbbells on your thighs, palms facing you. Pull your shoulder blades back and down, lift one dumbbell up in front of you to chest height. Slowly lower to thigh then lift the opposite arm. Repeat, alternating arms. For a harder version, lift both arms at the same time.

Technique tip: Brace your core to avoid momentum from your body.

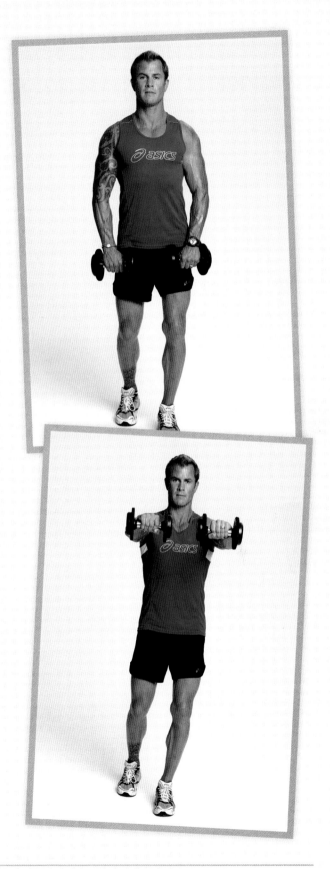

Dumbbell shoulder press

Sit using an upright bench to support your back or stand with feet hip width apart, and knees slightly bent. Hold dumbbells on your shoulders with palms facing forwards. Brace your stomach, press dumbbells up above your head until elbows are straight. Slowly lower and repeat.

Technique tip: Lift and lower dumbbells in a controlled fashion to avoid excess stress in the shoulder joint. Keep elbows slightly forwards of the body.

Variations: Incline dumbbell shoulder press. Do the shoulder press seated on an incline bench

Swiss ball dumbbell press. Do a shoulder press seated on the ball. Sit directly on top of the ball with knees at right angles, feet flat and abs braced.

Technique tip: Be sure to brace your abs to keep the ball still as you do the exercise — this increases the activation of the core muscles dramatically and stabilises the hips to form a strong foundation to lift from.

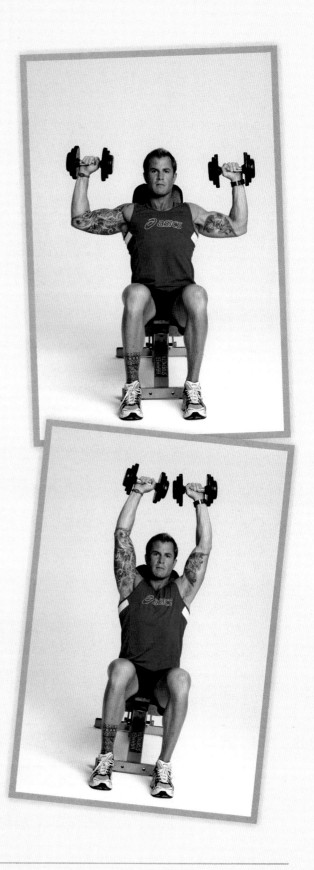

Machine shoulder press

Sit with your back against the seat, feet flat on the floor. Grip the handles. Press up, lower and repeat.

Technique tip: Avoid pushing your back into the seat; maintain natural curvature of the spine. Avoid craning the neck forwards.

Dumbbell side raises

Stand with feet hip width apart, one foot forwards, one foot back, and knees slightly bent. Hold dumbbells by your sides with palms facing in. Maintaining a slight bend in your elbows, lift the dumbbells up to the sides, keeping in line with your shoulders. Lift to shoulder height, giving your shoulder blades a slight squeeze at the top. Slowly lower and repeat.

Technique tip: Don't lift arms past parallel to the floor; lifting any higher places unnecessary strain on the shoulders.

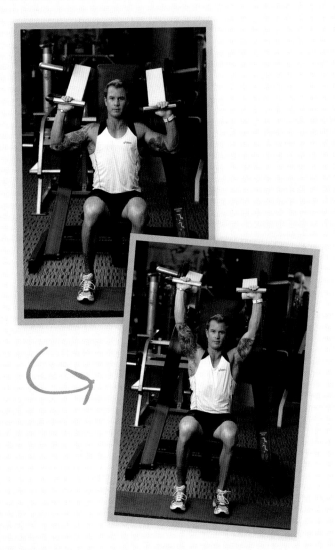

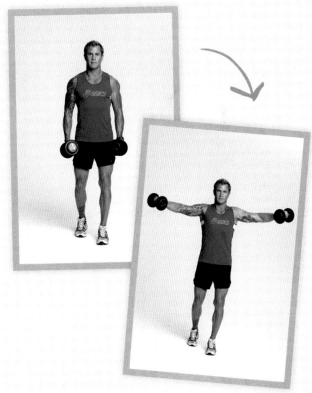

Body part: Legs/glutes

The glutes (gluteus maximus) spans your entire backside and is a mighty muscle, responsible for many movements such as walking, running and even getting up out of your chair. The leg muscles consist of your thigh muscles and lower leg muscles. On the front of your thigh are your quadriceps ('quads'), on the back of your thigh are your hamstrings ('hamis'), on the inner thigh are your adductor muscles. Below the knee, sit your calf muscles: gastrocnemius and soleus.

Dumbbell squats

Stand with feet shoulder width apart, holding dumbbells by your hips (to help with technique, you can place a bench behind you). Slowly sit down letting the dumbbells slide down over your hips (if using a bench your butt should barely touch it), then stand up. Maintain the natural curve of your spine and keep your chest up ('proud'), eyes looking forwards. Keep your weight grounded through the middle of your feet and heels. Do not use blocks under heels. Keep your knees aligned with the direction of your toes.

Technique tip: Do not bend your knees forwards over the line of your toes.

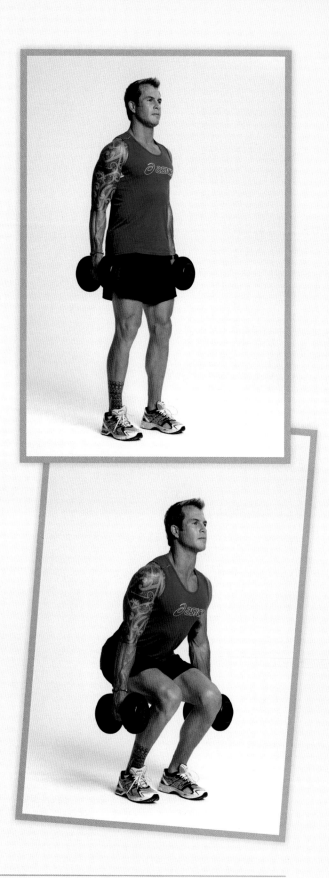

Smith machine squats

Scoop your neck underneath the bar. Position the bar across the top of your upper shoulders. Stand up and unlatch the lever. Steady your feet hip width apart, lower the bar and squat down as if you were sitting on a chair, push back up until your legs are straight, but don't lock your knees into position, and repeat.

Technique tip: Place feet slightly forwards of bar to avoid knees travelling too far past your toes.

Variation: Do barbell squats if you don't have access to a Smith machine.

Barbell squats

Do a squat, positioning the barbell (or Olympic bar) across the top of your shoulders. To position the barbell, get someone to place it across your shoulders and make sure you've got a firm hold before they let go or, preferably, use a squat rack. You can also do these in front of a bench to begin, to help get the squat action right.

Technique tip: Place the bar on the 'meaty' bit across the top of your shoulders, not the bony bit in your neck.

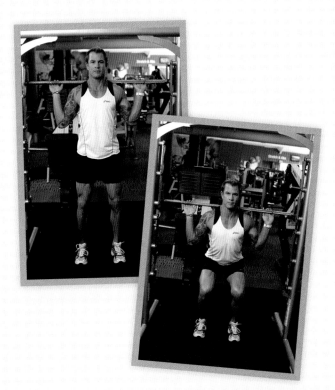

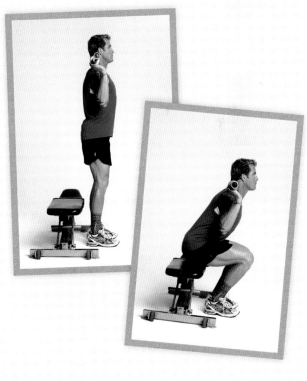

Lying leg curl

Face the bench and stand between the bench and the pads where you will hook your feet under. Lie face down so that your knees sit on the edge of the bench and your lower legs above your heels sit on the pads. Grasp the handles. Lift your feet (pads) to meet your backside by bending your knees, slowly lower and repeat.

Technique tip: Keep chest pressed down firmly on the bench to avoid excess strain on the lower back.

Leg press

Place feet hip width apart on the platform, knees in line with feet. Keep your back pressed against the seat, push the platform off the rack and turn the handles to release the rack. Straighten your legs (knees still slightly bent) — this is your start position. Lower the foot platform in a slow and controlled manner, keeping feet flat. Push the foot platform forwards until legs are straight (do not lock the knees into position), lower and repeat.

Technique tip: Do not bend your knees any further than 90 degrees to avoid placing too much pressure on the joint.

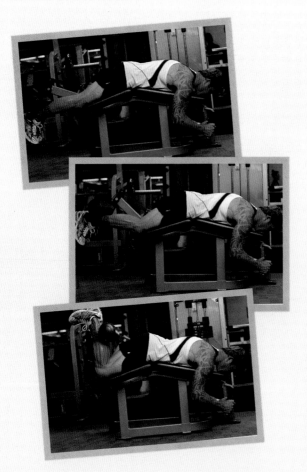

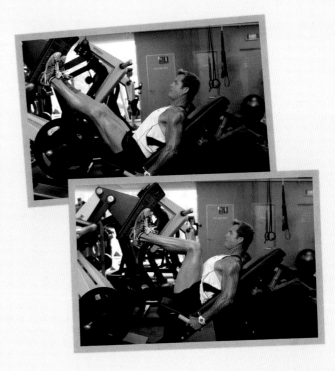

Leg extension

Sit on the seat and hook your feet underneath the foot pads. Lift your feet up until your knees are almost straight, slowly lower and repeat.

Technique tip: Avoid locking the knees into position.

Walking dumbbell lunges

Stand with feet hip width apart, holding dumbbells by your sides. Take a long step forwards with one leg, placing your foot in line with your hip. Bend your knees until your front thigh is parallel (or almost parallel) with the ground, and your back knee almost touches the ground. Push back up, bringing the back foot to meet the front one, pause, or step straight through this time taking the opposite leg forwards. Lunge and repeat continuing forwards. (Do not place your feet to the centre; position your feet as if along parallel train tracks.)

Technique tip: Never bend the front knee past the line of your ankle to avoid placing strain on the knee.

Variations: Do standing lunges on the spot.

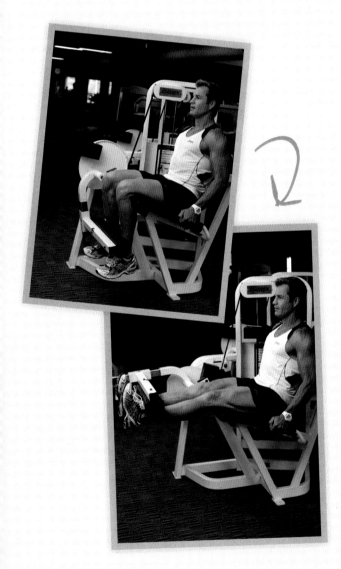

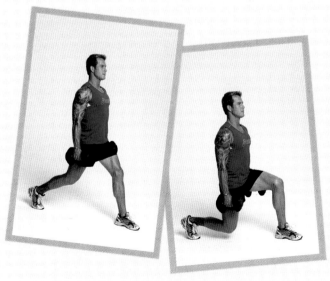

Romanian dead lift

Stand in front of the barbell with feet shoulder width apart. Keep your back upright, squat down and grasp the bar in a pronated grip with hands positioned just outside your feet. Look forwards, pull shoulders back and down, and tip from your hips only so that your back maintains its natural curve but doesn't bend (think long, flat back). Keeping your back upright and the bar very close to your shins and legs, pull the bar up as you stand up. Squeeze your backside in and thrust your hips slightly forwards on the way up. Slowly lower the bar back down, tipping from the hips, and keeping the bar close to your shins. Stop when you feel a good stretch in your hamstrings (usually just below your knee). Remember to stop before you round your back.

Technique tip: Ensure you have correct technique when doing this exercise; get a professional to supervise your technique at first.

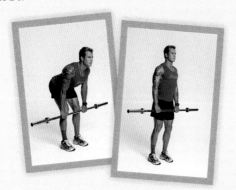

Dumbell dead lift

Do a dead lift (see Romanian dead lift) holding dumbbells with palms facing your shins.

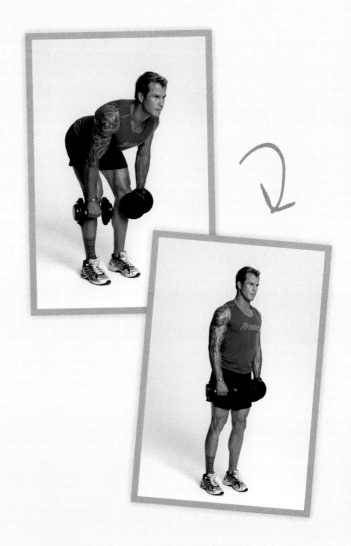

Smith machine lunges

Stand in the machine, position the barbell across your shoulders with one foot forwards and flat on the ground, back foot up on your toes and knees slightly bent. Lunge. Repeat on the other leg.

Technique tip: Position the front foot so that the front knee doesn't pass over the line of the ankle on the front foot.

Dumbbell step-ups

Step onto a sturdy bench, holding dumbbells by your side. Bring the other knee up. Step back down and repeat, leading with the same leg. Do the required reps and repeat, leading with the opposite leg.

Technique tip: Start out on a bench as high as halfway up your shin. As you get stronger, use a higher bench. Bench should never be higher than your knee to avoid straining the knee.

Variation: Alternate legs each time you step up.

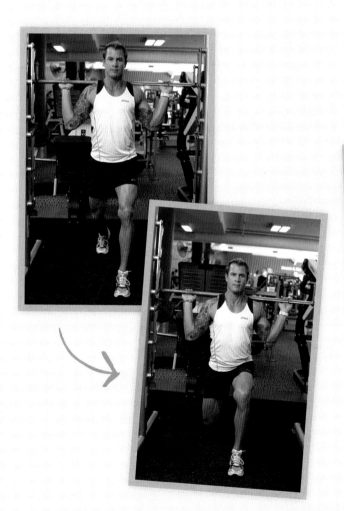

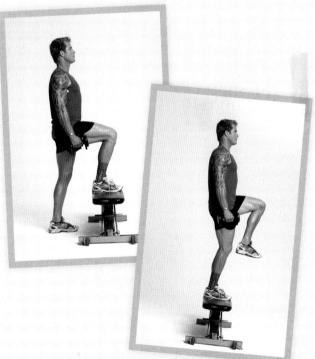

Standing calf raise

Stand with feet close together. Raise up on your toes, lower and repeat. Add weight in the form of holding dumbbells; positioning a barbell across your shoulders; doing the raises inside a Smith machine; or using a calf raise weight machine.

Technique tip: Squeeze right up on to your tiptoes to get the most out of the movement; the weight should primarily be on the big toe joints.

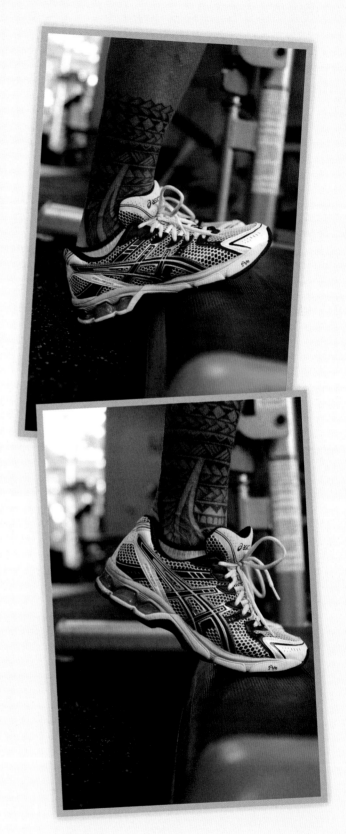

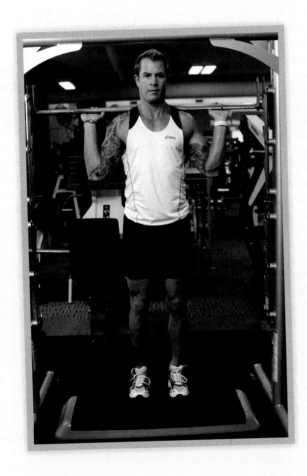

Body part: Abdominals (Abs)

Your stomach is made up of the rectus abdominis (main muscle running vertically down your stomach), the obliques (sit on each side of your stomach towards the waist) and the transverse abdominis or 'TA' (deepest muscle in the stomach often referred to as the postural muscle).

Crunch/sit-ups

Lie on the ground with knees bent, feet flat and hands on your thighs (for a harder version, fold your arms across your chest or place your hands behind your head with elbows pointing out). Use your abdominals to curl your upper body until your shoulder blades are off the ground, sliding your hands up your thighs, bringing your fingertips to your knees. Slowly lower to starting position and repeat.

Technique tip: Think 'crunch' (round out your back) rather than sit straight up.

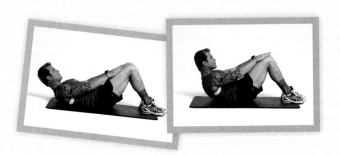

Oblique crunch

Lie on the ground with knees bent, feet flat. Place one hand behind your head, the other on your stomach and cross one foot over the other knee. Crunch up, bringing your elbow to meet the opposite knee and repeat. Do the same on the other side.

Technique tip: Beginners, keep one hand behind your head crunching towards the opposite knee, the other hand on the floor stretched out at 90 degrees to your body, pressing into the floor to help with the movement.

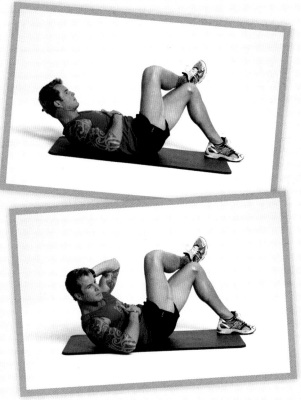

Bosu crunch

Complete a crunch lying over a bosu ball with knees bent and feet flat — this allows you to open your abs further than if you were on flat ground by giving you a greater range of motion. Your lower back should always be supported by the ball.

Technique tip: The closer your hips are to the front of the bosu the easier the exercise, with your backside sitting at the front of the bosu being the easiest version.

Swiss ball crunch

Using a Swiss ball provides a greater range of motion than a standard crunch. Sit on the ball with knees bent and feet flat. Carefully walk your feet forwards as you recline back onto the ball. Your hips should be sitting at the front of the ball and your lower back supported by the curve of the ball. Keeping the ball steady, with arms crossed on your chest or hands behind your head, crunch up. Slowly lower, keeping the ball still and your stomach muscles switched on, and repeat.

Technique tip: Keep your hips steady on the ball to anchor the movement.

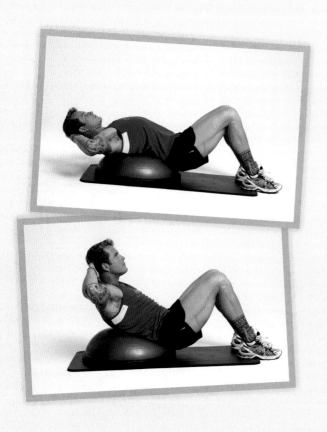

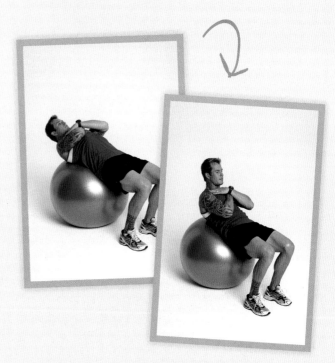

Reverse crunch

Lie flat on your back with hands by |your side, palms on the ground. Lift your legs off the floor and bend them at 90 degrees. Use your abdominals to lift your bottom off the floor, squeezing your pelvis towards your chest. Slowly lower to starting position and repeat.

For a harder version, straighten the legs and push feet up as you lift your backside up off the ground.

Technique tip: Always keep your 'belly button pulled in to your spine', breathe out as you contract. Avoid swinging the legs for momentum. Think rolling into a ball.

Incline reverse crunch

Lie on an incline bench with your head at the top of the bench and grab the top of the bench with both hands. Bend your knees and lift them up, keeping feet roughly in line with your knees. Contract your abdominals, lift your backside slightly off the bench and bring your knees towards your chest — think rolling into a ball — and repeat.

Technique tip: Lift and lower legs slowly to avoid momentum.

Variations: *Incline crunch.* Lie on an incline bench with your head at the bottom, feet hooked under pads at the top; complete a crunch as normal.

Incline oblique crunch. Lie on an incline bench with your head at the bottom, feet hooked under pads at the top; complete an oblique crunch as normal.

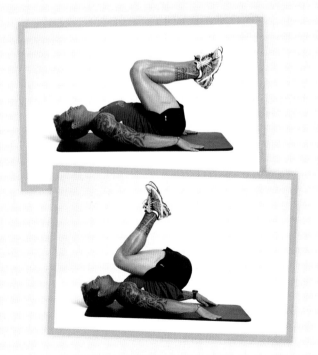

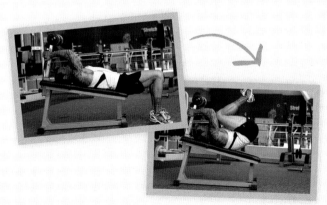

Bicycle crunch

Lie flat on the ground with your hands behind your head. Bend your knees at a 90 degree angle and lift your feet off the ground. Raise your shoulders off the ground and bring your left elbow to your right knee, hold for a second and really squeeze your abdominals, then bring your right elbow to your left knee and so on — continue the 'bicycling' action.

Technique tip: Keep your abs braced and aim to get your elbow to touch your knee.

Plank

Lie face down and then prop yourself up on your elbows under your shoulders, legs straight out behind you, feet together, resting on your toes. Keep your body long, maintaining the natural curve of your spine, squeeze and brace your abdominals, and hold for as long as you can.

Technique tip: Pull your belly button in towards your spine, don't hunch your shoulders or let your backside drift up into the air.

Variation: Place knees on the ground for a modified plank, so your torso makes a diagonal line from head to heel.

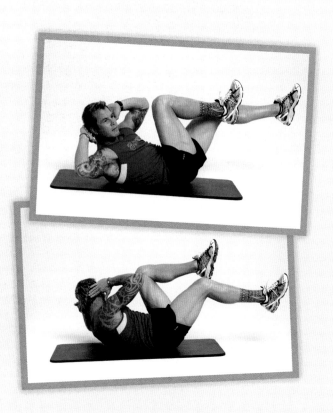

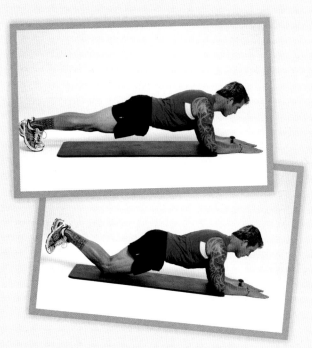

V-sits

Lie on the ground with arms and legs outstretched. Crunch up, bringing your hands to meet your toes in the middle of the 'V' and repeat.

Technique tip: Start off with a shorter range of movement and work your way up to touching your hands and toes.

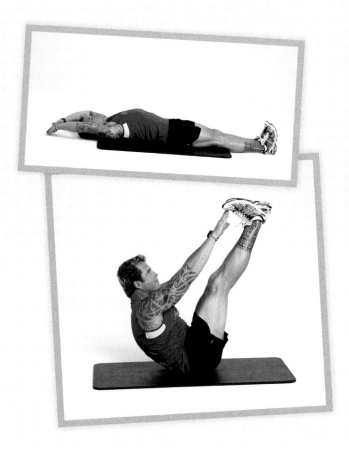

Flab to abs? Not quite

Sit-ups are the most overdone exercise, universally. Doing 1000 crunches a day will not deliver the six-pack you've dreamed about if there's excess body fat covering your abs! Every human has a six-pack waiting to be uncovered, but a visible, well-defined tummy is always a direct result of low body fat, not countless crunches. For most men, the level of body fat you'd have to reach to get those ripped abs is generally below 9 per cent! So forget those 'Flab to abs' gadgets and promises; fix your diet and do cardio to shed body fat, 'rip up' and unveil your very own washboard!

The stretches

Stretches can be done as part of your warm up and/or cool down. Be sure to do a few minutes of light cardio activity or a few sets on a light weight when resistance training before stretching as part of your warm up. Hold each stretch for 30 seconds–1 minute

Standing quad stretch

Stand or hold onto something, such as the back of a chair, for balance. Holding onto your ankle pull your right foot to your backside (as far as you can) with your right hand. Hold and repeat on the other leg. Keep your knees together and push your hips forwards.

Standing hamstring stretch

Stretch out one foot (or place up on a bench or chair), keeping your front knee straight. Keep your back upright, lean forwards from your hips until you feel the stretch down the back of your thigh on the straight leg. Hold and repeat on the other leg.

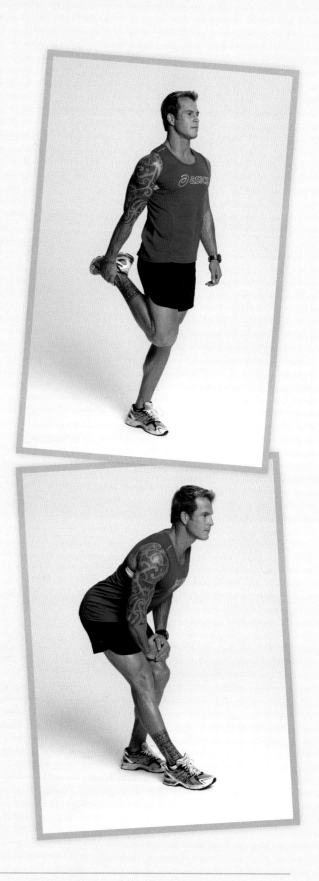

Hip flexor stretch

Kneel down (kneel on a rolled up towel or exercise mat if you need to relieve knee pressure) on one knee and place the other leg in front of you with your foot flat; both knees bent at a 90-degree angle. Tuck your backside under and lean forwards until you feel a stretch down the front of the hip of the leg behind you. Hold and repeat on the other leg.

Calf 'runners' stretch

Place both hands on a wall with arms stretched. Place one foot forwards and one foot back hip width apart; toes pointing forwards and both heels on the ground. Lean in to the wall, keeping the back knee straight until you feel a stretch in your calf muscle. Hold and repeat on the other leg. Repeat the same stretch on both legs, this time with a bent knee on the back leg, placing your weight through the back heel, to target your Achilles tendon area.

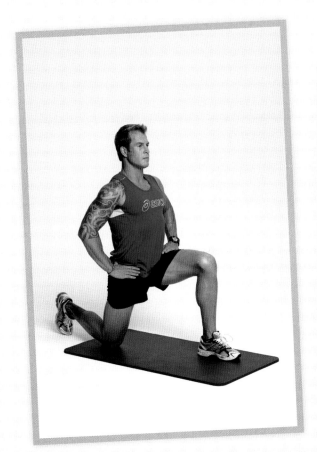

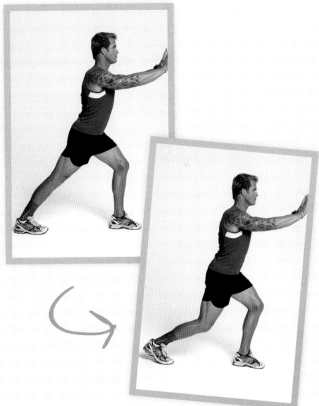

Chest stretch

Stand inside a door frame with elbows flexed at 90 degrees and hands on either side of the door frame. Lean forwards, keeping your shoulders pulled back until you feel your chest stretch, and hold.

Variation: If you don't have a door: Interlock your fingers behind your back. Elevate your hands and pull your shoulder blades together until you feel it stretch your chest.

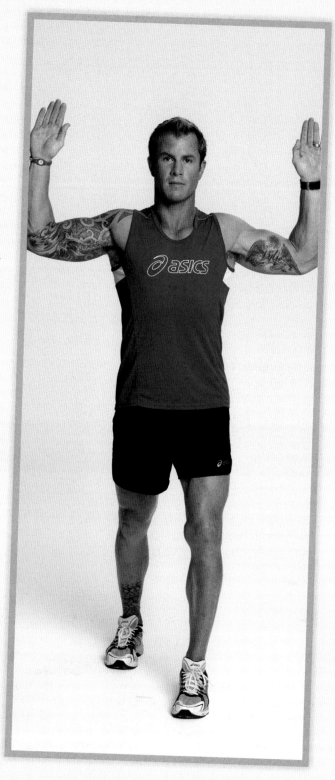

Back stretch

Interlock hands together in front of you
and turn your palms towards the floor.
Round your back then slowly raise your
arms while pushing your hands away from
your body until you feel a stretch in your
upper back and shoulders. Hold.

Triceps stretch

Stretch your right arm up towards the
ceiling. Bend your elbow so your hand
is behind your neck. Grab your right elbow
with your left hand and gently push
your right elbow down. Repeat with
the other arm.

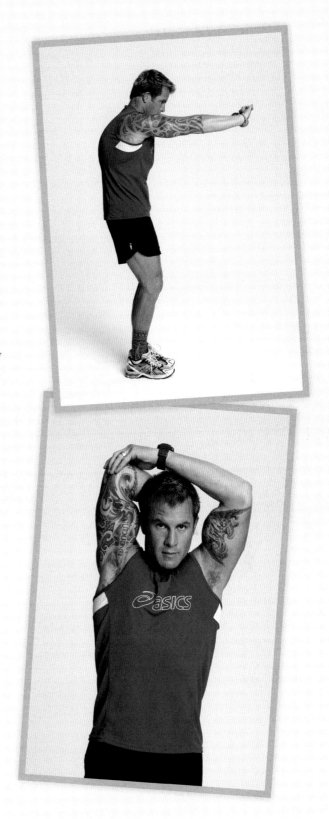

Exercise outside the gym

While seriously sculpting and shaping your body is best done with gym equipment, there are some great replacement exercises when training outside of the gym or when combining resistance exercises with your cardio workouts to make a circuit.

Upper body exercises

Push-ups *(works chest, as well as front shoulders)*: Push-ups can be done anywhere, anytime. Place hands shoulder width apart, fingers facing forwards, legs out straight behind you and the balls of the feet on the ground. Keep your body in a straight line from head to heel (no sagging stomachs or hunched shoulders). Lower your chest towards the floor by bending your elbows outwards until your chest is a fist-width off the ground. Push back up and repeat.

Variations: *Modified push-ups (easier)*: Even beginners can start on their toes, just limit the depth. You may start only being able to lower a couple of centimetres as you get stronger go a little deeper. But people with injuries should do modified push-ups – simply place your knees on the ground to make a straight diagonal line from head to knees. Complete the push-up as normal.

Decline push-ups (harder): Place feet up on a log/ bench to do push-ups

Tricep push-ups (targets triceps): Use a narrow grip and bend elbows close in to the body.

Bench dips *(works triceps)*: Do tricep dips (see page 202) off a log, park bench or step.

Outdoor chin-ups *(works back)*: Use a sturdy tree branch or a chin-up bar in an outdoor workout station to do chin-ups (see page 195).

Resistance band lat pull down *(works back)*: Toss a band over a tree branch and do lat pull downs.

Resistance band seated row *(works back)*: Wrap a band around a post and do seated row.

Resistance band bicep curl *(works biceps)*: Stand on the band and curl up.

Lower body exercises (works legs and glutes)

Bench squats: Do squats (see page 207) in front of a park bench using just your body weight or hold a medicine ball (harder) or piggy back a partner (advanced) as you squat.

Squat jumps: Perform a squat, touch the ground with one hand then propel yourself vertically with both feet leaving the ground and aim for height. Land softly into another squat and repeat, this time jumping up leading with the other hand.

Frog jumps: Do a squat jump, but instead propel yourself forwards and aim for distance.

Walking lunges: Do walking lunges (see page 198) with just your body weight or holding a medicine ball (harder) or uphill (harder).

Standing lunges: Step forwards, lunge, bring front foot to meet back foot and repeat.

Variations: *Alternating lunges:* Alternate legs each time you step forwards and back from your lunge.

Reverse lunges: Step back into the lunge instead of forwards.

Lunge jumps *(also called split squats or plyometric lunges)*: Jump up out of a standing lunge, change legs, lunge, jump up out of lunge, change legs, lunge and so on.

Step-ups: Do step-ups (see page 211) onto a bench or log with just your body weight or hold a medicine ball as you step-up (harder) or do a step-up with a knee repeat lift so the bottom foot stays planted on the ground as you step up on the same leg (harder), or jump up and down step or log (advanced).

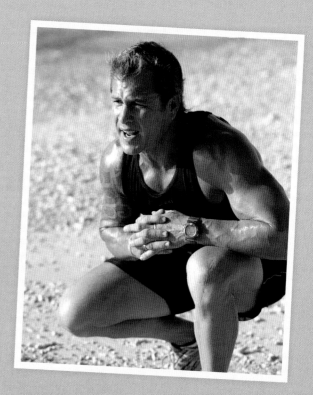

Core exercises
(works abdominals)

Varied crunches: Do all variations as described on pages 213–216.

Total body exercises

Burpees: Place your hands on the ground, push legs behind you, bring knees into chest, jump back up and repeat.

Lizard crawl: Walk along with your body close to and facing the ground on your hands and feet.

Commando crawl: Lie face down on the ground. Pull yourself along the ground using bent elbows.

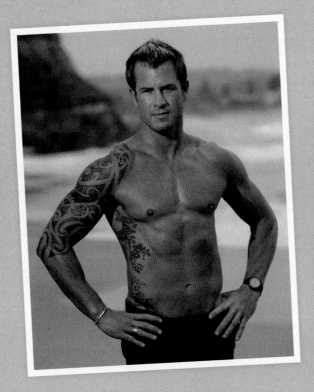

Ode to the outdoors

I love a good workout in the great outdoors. Here are some awesome outdoor sessions.

Time/Task Intervals

Time: Repeat as many sets as you can of 10 push-ups, 10 crunches, 10 burpees followed by a 400-metre sprint, as you can in 15 minutes. Use your imagination to construct exercises and distances. For best results repeat the same sequence for 5–6 workouts, each session aim to complete more rounds.

Task: Repeat 5 sets of 10 squat jumps, 10 v-sits (see page 217 for how to do a v-sit), 10-metre frog jumps, 10-metre lizard crawl followed by 100-metre sprint up and back (a total 200 metres). Use your imagination to construct exercises and distances. For best results repeat the same sequence for 5–6 workouts, each session aim to complete the 5 sets in a shorter time.

Tabata Intervals

Select a minimum of 5 exercises (you can do up to 10). Each exercise is performed flat out for 20 seconds followed by a 10 second rest, repeat this 4 times (total time: 2 minutes). Rest 1 minute, then start the next exercise in the same fashion. Try to match the number of reps you did in your first 20-second bout, each of the four times.

Pyramid

Set up a square (say half a football field). Select one exercise from each group of exercises (body part) to do in each corner. Start in one corner with 10 reps of an upper body exercise, walk/run/sprint to the next corner, perform 10 reps of a lower body exercise, walk/run/sprint to the next corner, do a total body exercise, walk/run/sprint to the next corner, do a core exercise.

Repeat, the whole sequence, this time doing 12 reps, then 14 reps, then 16, then 18, all the way to 20 reps!

Beginners start with lower reps, say 5, then increase by 1 rep until you get to 10. The fitter you get the higher in reps you go!

Simply sets

Just like weight training in the gym select one exercise for each body part. For example, push-ups (chest), resistance band lat pull down (back), squats (legs), resistance band bicep curl (biceps), tricep dips and plank.

Perform 3 sets of 5-15 reps (depending on your fitness). This can be done as a circuit, body part to body part, no rest, or 3 sets of push-ups with 30 second rest, then move to lat pull down, and so on.

Progress by striving for more reps or choosing a more challenging exercise.

Awesome outdoor training tools

- Resistance band
- Medicine ball
- Focus pads and boxing mitts
- ViPR Bars (a weighted tube that can be used for just about any form of resistance training or agility drill; a versatile and handy tool)
- Park benches, logs and steps

PART 4: KEEP IT UP!

You've learned the ins and outs of weight loss and got the tools you need to lose weight and rebuild your body and life. Now how do you apply all of this information, incorporate it into your daily life and keep up the momentum? Through balance, maintaining energy and staying true to one important mantra: Never, ever, EVER give up!

Chapter 10:
Balance it UP

You need to create the necessary time and space to look after yourself, train, prepare healthy meals and be the best version of yourself. This requires a balance between work and life.

Work doesn't just involve those who pay taxes — stay-at-home mothers, carers, students and volunteers can all be putting in the same amount of hours as those on the payroll. While some people's motives for work are in line with important values, such as helping others and providing for your family, no matter what your motivation, if you devote too much time to work and not enough time to your life, you won't be able to take care of you — your weight, health, and happiness. And unless you take care of and put some time into yourself (this isn't a selfish act), you will never be at your best.

You've got to strike a balance between what you do for others and what you do for YOU. To do this, you need to weigh up your priorities.

Make health and happiness a priority

Health and happiness go hand in hand; you can't have one without the other. You must value health and happiness as a top priority in order to make room for the things in your life that make you healthy and happy, such as time spent with family, training, cooking nutritious meals or getting a massage.

Let's talk about your definition of happiness for a moment.

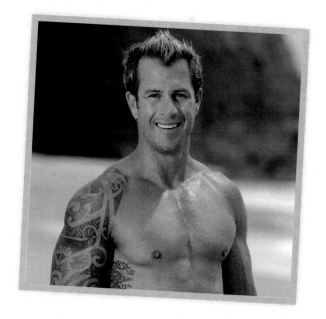

What does happiness mean to you?

What's your earliest happy memory? For most, it's associated with family such as holidays at Grandma's, Christmas day with the whole family, playing with a sibling, Dad teaching you to ride a bike, Mum taking you to dancing lessons.

To all parents and future parents I challenge you with this question: *What will your child's earliest happy memory be … will you be in it?*

Are you spending too much time working and striving for material possessions? Are you so overworked, unhealthy, tired and drained that you don't have the energy to be actively involved in your kids' lives?

Now if you're working so hard to provide for your family, working two jobs to keep your family above the poverty line, if you're doing this to genuinely keep food on the table, more power to you and your kids will respect and remember that with gratitude. But if your endless hours spent at work is a purely self-indulgent pursuit — for example, I have to work more because when I drop the kids off at the most prestigious (and probably most expensive) private school I've got to be

in the latest BMW, wearing the latest designer shades, and my kids have to wear labels, and have the most expensive gear — if that's where your head is at, you have to take a look at your priorities because this is not what kids remember and appreciate; kids remember and appreciate time with their family — memories!

The same is true for those who devote all of their time working for others, as a stay-at-home mum, a carer or volunteer. While your motives may not be self-indulgent, if you give over all of your time to your kids or those you're helping, they too will suffer in the long run, because if you don't look after yourself you can't properly look after someone else. You will get burnt out, your health and energy levels will suffer and you won't be able to give your all to your kids and loved ones. It's better to spend that little bit less time, but quality time where you're happy and in the moment, than be with them all of the time where you're unhappy, snappy and not in the moment.

Many mothers are desperately trying to 'keep up appearances', wearing themselves thin, thinking they're doing the right thing by selflessly helping everyone else and taking on everyone's problems. I see it all the time on *The Biggest Loser*: female contestants coming to the show defining themselves as 'the perfect mothers and wives'. But they have really just hidden themselves away from life – they were just existing, surviving the day, not living – and every family member knew it. There were no family holidays, shopping together, outings, going to the beach, just perfectly ironed clothes and spotless houses. Their entire families were suffering. They would lose a staggering amount of weight but the physical changes paled into insignificance compared to the emotional and mental transformations. Now, these women and their families are rocking this life, living every moment, with no regrets.

'You can't e
complete h
unless you
complete h

perience
ppiness
experience
alth.'

Shannan Ponton

The 'I'll be happy when ...' syndrome

How much of your happiness is dependent on getting something or somewhere?

Many people think they'll be happy when they arrive at some place other than now. Take, for example, someone in an unhappy relationship ... 'I'll be happy when we get engaged', turns into 'I'll be happy when we get married' turns into 'I'll be happy when we move out of this small apartment' turns into 'I'll be happy when we have kids to fill our big house' turns into 'I'll be happy when we can buy a brand-new family car' turns into 'I'll be happy when we can buy a better house in a better area' turns into 'I'll be happy when the kids finish school so we can travel'. All of a sudden you die, having wished away 15, 20, 30, 40 years of your life because you were always pinning your happiness on something in the future. (Sorry to sound like a downer, but remember, life is not a dress rehearsal; you don't get to do it again.)

Waiting for happiness to come in the form of a partner, house, baby, car or job means you're linking your definition of happiness to people and possessions; that you're trying to fill a hole inside of you with things that exist outside of you.

When you get the external 'thing', it may provide temporary relief and momentary happiness, but it doesn't last because you're reliant on the next 'thing' to fill you up again.

The same is true for weight loss. Thinking you'll finally be happy when you lose the weight and reach that dress size you dream of, implies you'll only be happy when you reach a future destination. But if you embark on your weight-loss journey from the viewpoint of feeling good each and every day because you're taking steps to take care of yourself, you can start experiencing happiness right now — with every step you take, every healthy meal you eat, and every small goal you achieve along the way.

See the difference? 'Taking care of myself makes me happy' is very different to 'I'll be happy when I lose 40 kilograms'. 'Going for a walk each day makes me happy' is very different to 'I'll be happy when I'm fit'. A journey is not defined by reaching the destination; it's the sum of your experiences and what you learn along the way that makes the journey.

I went from being a very fat and sad housewife and mum to a person who loves life and is making the most of every opportunity. Having Shannan as my trainer, mentor and rock, and now very special friend, has been the most life-changing period of my life. Shannan unleashed the hidden me, stripped me back to my core, and then helped me to rebuild a better stronger and freer Lisa. I'm now an active participant in my children's lives, not just an observer, and feel I have been given an amazing, life-changing gift.

—Lisa Hose, 2010 Series of The Biggest Loser

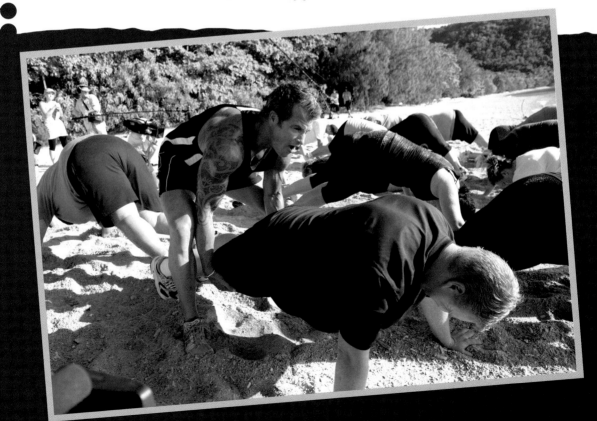

Weigh it up: effort versus benefit

An important part of sticking to your goals and program is positive self-talk. When your thoughts become negative such as 'I can't do this', 'It hurts too much', 'I want to give up', 'What's the use anyway?' — you need to weigh up the effort you're putting into it against the benefit you're getting out of it. Keep these two thoughts imprinted on your mind:

Pain versus Results
Commitment versus Rewards

Yes, training is hard and it hurts but the pain is short lived; the results last. Yes, achieving your weight-loss goal requires discipline and commitment which can be hard to maintain, but the rewards you're getting — a new body, health, self-confidence … getting your life back! — far outweigh the energy and effort of your commitment.

We've never had a contestant standing on the scales at the finale who doesn't say that every moment of pain and hard work was worth it. In that moment they feel so good and empowered, all the pain becomes a distant memory.

Tossing up the idea of surgery?

Losing masses of weight is an enormous task and may leave stretched skin in its wake. There are surgical options to assist both weight loss and the after-effects of weight loss such as stretched, saggy skin.

• Lapband surgery

Also called gastric banding involves the insertion of a band, much like a wristwatch, around the upper stomach to create a smaller stomach, which restricts the amount of food you can eat, helping you to feel full and satisfied with smaller amounts of food. It is generally only offered to people who have a BMI of 40 or more. But, like any procedure, it does carry associated risks such as nausea and vomiting, reflux and internal blockages.

In my opinion, in 99 per cent of times, surgery to help lose weight is an unnecessary risk. In all my time in the industry I have not seen a person who won't lose weight once they get their diet right and activity levels up. Any surgery to aid weight loss is not addressing the lifestyle habits that have and will continue to cause you to be overweight.

• Removal of excess skin

When you lose weight and fat the skin doesn't always retract back at the same rate as the weight loss. The skin is made up of fibres that get stretched with weight gain. When there is weight loss, these fibres don't always spring back into place, instead they may come back together slowly, retracting to a certain degree, but never fully. If this is the case, you may be left with excess skin that only surgery will get rid of. Common areas for excess skin removal are the chest (man boobs), inner thigh, triceps and stomach.

Having done everything to tighten up and tone saggy bits after massive weight loss, a person may still not like the appearance of their body, in this case getting plastic surgery can boost their self-image and self-esteem. For some plastic surgery is the final step in allowing them to feel 'normal'.

- Tummy tuck

One of the most common orders with weight loss is a flat, toned tummy. Unfortunately, for some people, no matter how many crunches they do they don't get that six-pack they thought they would as a result of losing weight. Instead, they're left with saggy, soft rolls of skin in their lower stomach. This is especially true for women struggling to get rid of their post-pregnancy bump. During pregnancy women can experience a separation of the main abdominal muscle (this occurrence is known as diastasis recti). Basically, the sides of the biggest muscle that runs down your stomach

(rectus abdominis) pull away from each other leaving a gap in the middle. If you have this condition you can usually feel a gap or space in the middle of your stomach just below your navel. While this occurrence isn't painful or harmful, the gap can get worse, leaving you with that flabby tummy you don't want.

The first line of action is to do abdominal exercises to help bring the muscles back together, particularly core abdominal exercises that strengthen the deep stomach muscle (called transverse abdominis) such as fitball sit-ups and Pilates. But if an intense core-training program coupled with fat loss doesn't produce the desired results, then surgery in the way of a tummy tuck might be a reasonable option for women who feel self-conscious about their stomach area.

When weighing up the pros and cons of surgery it's important to remember that you first need to do everything you can by way of diet and exercise, and only seek surgery as a last resort. Many people are misinformed about drugs and surgery, usually having unrealistic expectations of the results. Surgery can help but it has associated risks and side effects, and is not a magic pill. If you are considering surgery, be sure to research thoroughly, consulting with many plastic surgeons and only go with a fully qualified surgeon who you feel comfortable with.

By finding ways to enjoy your weight-loss journey, rather than thinking enjoyment will only come when your goal weight is reached, you'll be more likely to stick with the program. For example, if you enjoy working out because you are learning new skills, spending time with other people, getting out in the fresh air or learning to run, then you're more likely to reach your goal weight and maintain your exercise program once you've lost the weight.

Health and happiness is a daily practice, a mindset, that you can start living now. Break the victim mentality and start living 'happy'. It's up to you.

Getting the balance right

To get your work-life balance right, it's time to weigh-in again, only this time using your own personal set of 'health and happiness' scales.

On one side of the scales we're measuring what you want to get as a result of your output and effort (Work). Be honest with yourself: is it money, recognition, power, achievement, social standing, self-satisfaction? On the other side of the scales we're measuring what you want to give as a result of your input, to yourself and others (Life). This might be time with family, time with friends, quality relationships, time for yourself to recharge your batteries such as going to the gym, taking a walk, doing a weekly yoga class — anything that makes you feel good and revitalised.

I used to think I was bulletproof but my body has taught me otherwise, signalling to me that I have to sometimes slow down, rest and recover. 2010 was the year of international bad health for me! After 10 courses of antibiotics and not heeding the doctor's advice to rest (I took 'rest' as train for one hour a day instead of three!), I ended up with pneumonia. As soon as I recovered from that I tore my left medial ligament off the bone, three weeks prior to the start of filming for The Biggest Loser, which required surgery and intense physio so I could be right for the show. Next, my wife spotted a dark spot on my leg, which I was totally unaware of, when we were honeymooning in Bali; she made an appointment right then and there from the beach for as soon as I got back — 15 stitches later I had a malignant melanoma cut out that was 0.6mm deep (1 mm and it's in your blood). I'll forever be defined by 0.4mm and forever in debt to my wife, who quite literally saved my life! The lesson I learned from all this is don't be ignorant to your body's messages — listen and take time out when you need to.

If you load the scales up on the 'work' side (what you're trying to get from life), the 'life' side (what you want to give to life) quickly gets incredibly light and suffers as a consequence. If you work furiously on one side to get what you want — I want money, I want power, I want a new wardrobe, I want recognition … I want, I want, I want — you'll have little to no time to give to yourself and health.

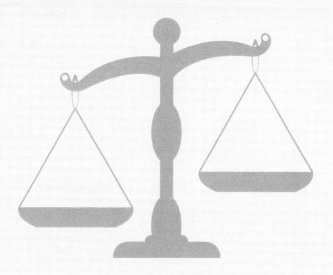

Manipulate the variables on either side of the scales according to what's important to you (hint: making time to exercise, eat and sleep well, and take care of yourself is considered important!). Assess what things on the work side you can take away to reduce your load in order to allow some time to do the things that will give you a good quality of life — more time with family and friends, and more time spent improving your health, weight, and wellbeing.

Work: What things do I genuinely need to do for work?

Life: What things do I need to do to be healthy and happy?

As you take things away from the work side of the scales you'll come up with all sorts of excuses and justifications as to why you have to work so much, such as 'My boss is increasing the workload', 'My wife really wants a new diamond ring', 'My kids really need the latest sports shoe', 'My family needs me to do everything for them'. This is where you'll need to be strong, take back control and tip your personal set of scales in your favour.

Once you've got the balance right for *you*, and created the necessary time and space to live a balanced, happy, healthy life, you're going to need the energy to keep it up.

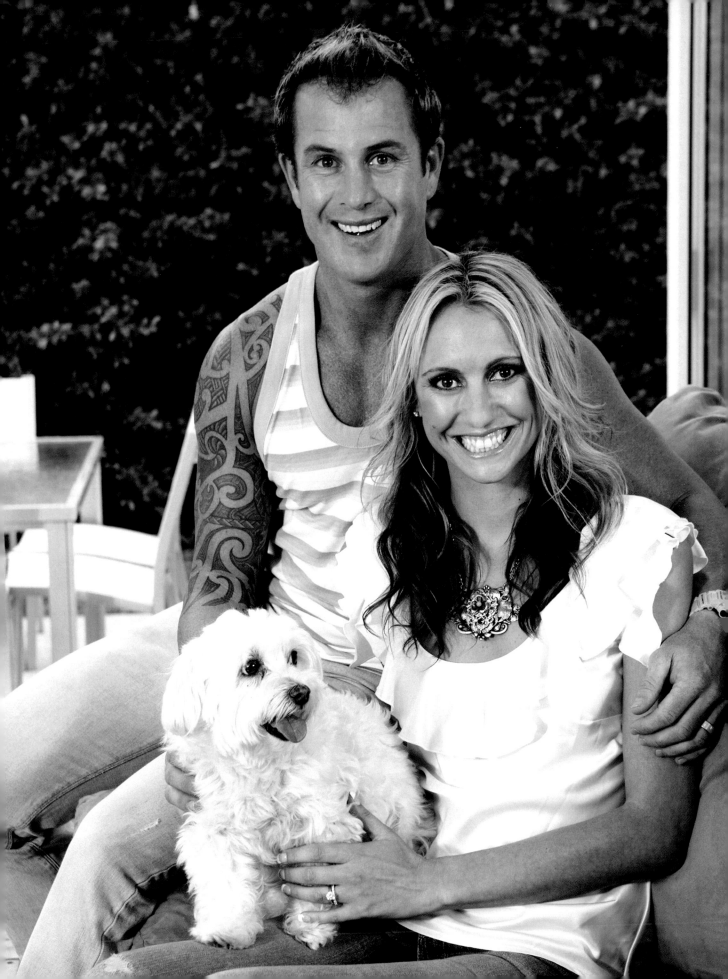

Chapter 11:
Charge UP

If you're going to make changes in your life and radically transform the way you think, eat, exercise and live, you're going to need the energy to do it.

Being too tired is a common complaint (excuse) that stands in the way of doing the work required to lose weight — that is, workout and eat well.

Many people seem to slump in energy once it hits 2 p.m. And that's when they justify that they need a bag of jelly beans or a chocolate bar to pick their energy up and get them through the afternoon.

Eating a chocolate or lollies or any other type of sugary food will not pep you up. It might provide a quick boost but the energy rush is short lived. Remember Blue Team Philosophy number 4, 'What goes up must come down'? When blood sugar goes up quickly, it quickly comes back down — leaving you flat and tired again. (Not to mention these types of foods are potential stored energy that if not burnt up will get stored as fat.)

There are 240 volts of energy running through the average electrical power point found at home and work. When you're tired and lacking in energy, you don't go and stick your finger into the electrical socket

for a 'pick me up' because it's the wrong type of energy. It's still energy but it has disastrous effects on your body. Sticking sugar and junk into your body is the same story; it's the wrong type of energy and has disastrous effects on your body — weight gain, elevated sugar in the blood, diabetes, and fatigue to name a few side-effects.

Stop believing that if you're tired you can eat some sugary, calorie-laden carbohydrate to give you energy. It doesn't and will make you fat! And, while you're at it, stop the myth (excuse) that you're too tired to exercise.

Exercise plus healthy food GIVES you energy.

Let's look at some simple ways to elevate your energy levels each day so you can never use the 'I'm too tired to cook/train/go for a walk/chop vegies …' excuse ever again!

Energy boosters

There are many ways to boost your energy that don't involve carbs, caffeine, chocolate or the couch! Try these.

Switch sleepy foods for energy foods

Food plays an important role in energy. Most people automatically think of eating carbohydrates when they need energy, but when carbs are broken down serotonin is released, causing you to feel slower and sleepier!

Also, the types of carbs people tend to reach for to boost their energy are processed sugars and starches — that muffin or doughnut with that mid-morning coffee, those lollies and chocolate bars in the afternoon. Once digested these foods will drastically spike blood sugar levels, causing your body to produce excess insulin and end up dropping your blood sugar to a lower level, making you feel even more tired and lower in energy.

If you're looking to boost your energy in the afternoon, cut out the processed sugars and starches for lunch and have protein and salad, and grab a high-protein snack in the afternoon such as a low-fat yoghurt or tin of tuna. Not only will this give you energy for the afternoon but will help you lose weight, feel lighter, think clearer and concentrate better.

Seek out success

Achievement creates energy to inspire further achievement. It's called the success snowball effect. You know the saying, 'If you want something done, give it to a busy person.' That busy person is always going to be energised, on top of it, efficient and will get the job done. Be inspired to achieve and you'll have the energy to keep achieving.

Surround yourself with positive people

Take a look at the people you surround yourself with. You don't want to be spending a lot of time around negative friends, the kind that when you call them up the conversation goes something like this:

How are you?
'Oh, I'm pretty tired.'

So what's been happening?
'Not much.'

Did you train today?
'Nah, didn't train, I was too tired.'

So what else has been happening?
'Don't know. Not much.'

What did you do on the weekend?
'Just took it easy.'

People like this will suck the energy right out of you! They're literally energy vampires! Where possible, limit your time with energy vampires and spend more time with positive people. If interactions like this are unavoidable, be very aware of your own energy when you speak to and spend time with these people so as not to get dragged into their low energy state.

Remember: who you spend time with you become. People's energy influences your energy and vice versa. I highly recommend breaking free of chronic perpetual energy vampires altogether!

Surround yourself with a panel of experts

You've got to be on the right track in order to get results because when you're not on the right track, your energy levels will suffer. The fish that's swimming with the current is going to have far more energy than the fish that's swimming against the current.

By surrounding yourself with a panel of experts, both professional and personal, you have constant compasses to keep you on the right track.

If you want to know about willpower and determination you probably don't want to ask your mate who has tried and failed to quit smoking 10 times because he's not going to know much about it. If you want to know about relationships, you want to talk to one of your friends in a long-term, fulfilling relationship; you don't want to talk to the person who's had a string of dysfunctional relationships or just got divorced because they're probably going to give you subjective, bad advice.

The same is true for diet, exercise and weight loss. Surround yourself with friends and professionals who know what it takes to get results — personal trainers, gym instructors, diet coaches, people who have successfully lost weight, gym members who have kept up a three-times-a-week commitment to the gym for the past 10 years.

Choose real friends

Friends who are honest — who tell you your haircut doesn't suit you, that your outfit is not very flattering, that your health is suffering and you're putting on weight — are a must. Because keeping it real and living in truth is essential for energy. Real friends, who are good sounding boards, are going to lift you up, not bring you down. Also, be sure to choose friends who give as well as take. An imbalance in energy will leave you depleted. You want friends that contribute to your life as you contribute to theirs; friends who put energy back into you so you walk away feeling good after spending time with them.

Channel your energy

Stop telling stories with your face and body language. Instead, put on your best poker face. If training hurts, you don't have to emphasise it by grimacing and contorting your face, instead, put that energy into your muscles, get in the zone, and get on with your training. If you don't feel up to doing something but you have to do it, don't slump your shoulders and moan and groan — hard'n up, pull your shoulders back, sit up straight, quit whining, shift your energy into the task at hand and get on with it. You'll be amazed at how such a simple thing as changing your body language and face can instantly lift your energy levels.

Master your environment

A huge influence on energy is your environment. There's nothing worse than visiting, or even worse, living in, a dark, dank, dirty place that makes you unhappy. Make your environment happy and inspiring. Some ways you can do this:

- Open the blinds and let lots of light in.

- Get a few minutes of sunlight each day, to top up your Vitamin D levels, which play a crucial role in energy and mood.

- Put a vase of flowers in your space.

- Hang happy pictures of holidays and loved ones.

- Stick motivational quotes on your computer, bathroom mirror, car windscreen, fridge and pantry.

- Place a mirror in the room to create the effect of space and light.

- Implement some feng shui.

- Whatever it is that floats your boat and puts a smile on your face; just add some personal touches to create the place where you're spending most of your time — be it at work, your desk, home, your car — a positive environment.

Maintain a positive outlook

Tiredness is largely a state of mind. Even if you have a bad night's sleep, don't get up the next day and drag your ass around with your tired, whingey, whiney, complaints because you'll be dragging everyone else down with you. If you are tired, make the most of what you can with the day, keep positive and simply get on with it.

Get adequate sleep

Take responsibility for your sleep. Initiate set sleep patterns, burn lavender oils in your bedroom, don't watch TV just before bed, avoid caffeine late in the day — whatever aids a restful night's sleep. Also, find an amount of sleep that works for you — some executives who run multi-million dollar companies and many world leaders have reported only needing around 4 hours sleep a night, but this doesn't work for everyone, so take note of what amount of sleep allows you to function at your best.

People who get less than 6 hours' sleep a night are more likely to be overweight and suffer health complications, such as heart disease.

Take big belly breaths

You can live for weeks without food, days without water but only 3 minutes without oxygen! Oxygen is the catalyst your body needs for life energy, clear thinking and vitality. When we breathe efficiently we take in energy-giving oxygen and expel energy-depleting toxins. When we're stressed we tend to take short, shallow, chest breaths, which doesn't get the oxygen in needed to perform at our best. The same is true for when you get exhausted from intense physical exercise, we tend to bend over, which squashes our breathing pump, the diaphragm, and take short, shallow breaths from the chest. Instead, you need to stand or sit tall, take deep breaths from your belly, so as you breathe in your diaphragm and stomach expands, and as you breathe out your stomach comes back in. Always breathe in through the nose and out through the mouth. Be sure to take regular stops throughout your day to take a few big belly breaths as well as make sure you're breathing efficiently when working out to maximise the energy you need to train at your optimum.

Give to others

A common question I get asked is, 'Do I feel drained from the physical, mental and emotional strain of training and helping people?' Yes, my line of work can be draining, but for every bit of energy I put out, I get at least twice the amount of energy put back in. When I help someone achieve their goals and I see the look of self-satisfaction, pride and accomplishment on their faces, when I know I've played a hand in transforming and saving their life in every sense of the word the energy flows back in and recharges my soul.

I get such a buzz from seeing the results people get. I quite often run with my contestants or clients in fun runs, and at times 50 per cent slower than I could. But when they finish the race and they've completed their first fun run, to see the look on their faces when they cross the finish line and throw their arms up in the air, then turn around and give me the biggest hug, it's real and pure and puts me on as much of a high as they are. This is what I call riding the natural high of life.

Giving to others requires energy but the rewards you get in return recharge your batteries.

Look for ways to help and give back to others. If you're a boss or manager, why not look deeper than motivating factors such as your salary or status, and look for ways that you can impart the lessons and knowledge you've learned to help employees have a more fulfilling life? What about giving one of your employees who has been working too much and not spending enough time with their family, the weekend off to spend it with loved ones? The appreciation you'll get back will be ten-fold — in time, effort, work ethic and commitment. Giving back in these small and simple ways recharges your soul because you know that you've played a hand in helping someone's life.

Exercise, exercise and exercise!

The biggest key to changing your energy levels is exercise. I don't know anyone who finishes a workout and says, 'Gee, I wish I didn't do that.' EVERYBODY feels better after doing a workout. There are no losers in exercise. It's win-win: you look and feel better; you have more energy; you're out and about getting amongst it; you're not letting life pass you by; and you feel more positive because you're doing something for yourself.

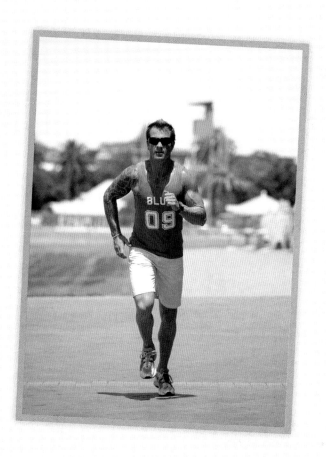

Shake things up!

Boredom is a huge energy zapper. It makes your motivation and your mood become stale. This also applies to your training and eating. Boredom can cause you to fall off the weight-loss wagon by losing interest and energy to keep up with your program. Sometimes you have to shake things up a little to keep your commitment in check and your weight loss cranking. Here are some tips for keeping your program varied and interesting:

- Take on a new physical challenge such as rockclimbing, surfing, bushwalking, mountain biking or even climbing a tree!

- Train in a different setting such as the park, beach, bush, footy stadium, netball courts, sand dunes.

- Try a new workout or exercise class. As you get fitter and lose weight you will build up more self-confidence to help you try new things.

- Do different exercises; there are countless exercises to choose from that work the same body part.

- Use different types of equipment such as a medicine ball, dumbbell, skipping rope, bosu ball and so on.

- Change the course of your walking, cycling or running path.

- Introduce your family and friends to your training and eating program; the social aspect does wonders for maintaining motivation (just make sure that when you exercise, you spend more time training than talking!).

- Experiment with different recipes using ingredients from your allowed list of foods.

- Adapt recipes from a variety of cookbooks and cuisines to make them low carb, low fat, high protein, low sugar, low salt.

- Plan weekly, monthly, and yearly rewards for achieving your weight-loss goals, such as a massage, clothes or a holiday. Incentive is a great motivator.

- Buy yourself some new clothes as you lose weight as a reward and self-esteem boost.

- Educate yourself by reading books, researching and talking to experts about new ways to eat healthy and exercise; there's plenty to learn and keep you interested!

- Set goals and challenges which inspire you such as entering a fun run, completing a marathon, your first triathlon, or training for a trek.

I recently did one of the best, most emotional and soul reviving, awe-inspiring things I've ever done: The Kokoda Trail. Reaching the plateau that is Isurava was one of the proudest moments of my life. The physical impact on the body from preparing and walking 'The Track' paled in comparison to the emotional impact. It was arduous, demanding and intense, with 5 a.m. starts and up to 9 hours of walking (sometimes climbing, clambering and sliding!), but so worth every ache, drop of sweat, blister and chafe!

Setting a trek to conquer is an incredible goal to keep your training and spirits motivated. The best way to prepare for a trek is to take long hikes, including steep hills, stairs or sand dunes, wearing the boots, socks and the backpack you intend to carry on your trek. Aim for around 30 minutes, three-four times a week, increasing by 10 minutes each week or so until you're doing around 90 minutes at a time. Adding weight gradually to your pack will also help to further your strength endurance. You can also prepare in the gym with exercises to strengthen your legs and core such as squats, lunges and step-ups with weights.

Jump UP for joy

When was the last time you literally jumped for joy? Not a too-cool-for-school 'yeah' or self-congratulatory pat on the back, but when you were actually so involved in what you were doing you got two feet off the ground and jumped up from a place of pure joy and passion?

I ask this question when I'm giving talks to groups of people. One of the most memorable answers I once received was from a guy who stood up and said, 'This is a little embarrassing, but the last time I jumped for joy was last Saturday when I beat my daughter at Wii Fit tennis.' Everyone laughed but I said that was fantastic. Here's a father who's playing a game with his daughter, not begrudgingly but with passion. He's not that guy thinking *Hurry up, darl, I've got to get to golf,* and saying 'Yeah good shot' in a half-hearted way because his mind isn't really there but where he wishes he was: out playing with his mates. In that moment he was committed, present and passionate, and was having a genuinely good time with his daughter.

So when was it? The last time you two-feet jumped for joy? Was it when your team won? When your child scored a goal? When your kids aced the ballet recital? When you got married? If you can't remember the time, take a good look at your life. Because without this type of joy in your life you'll most certainly run out of energy at some point.

If you can experience this sort of joy on a regular basis it means you're tapped into life's energy.

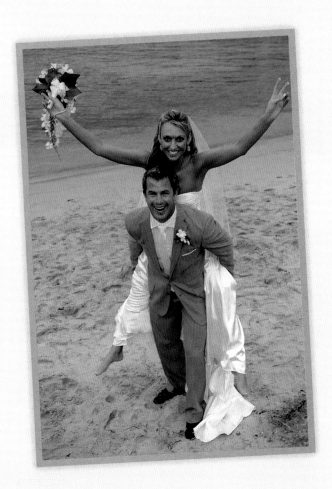

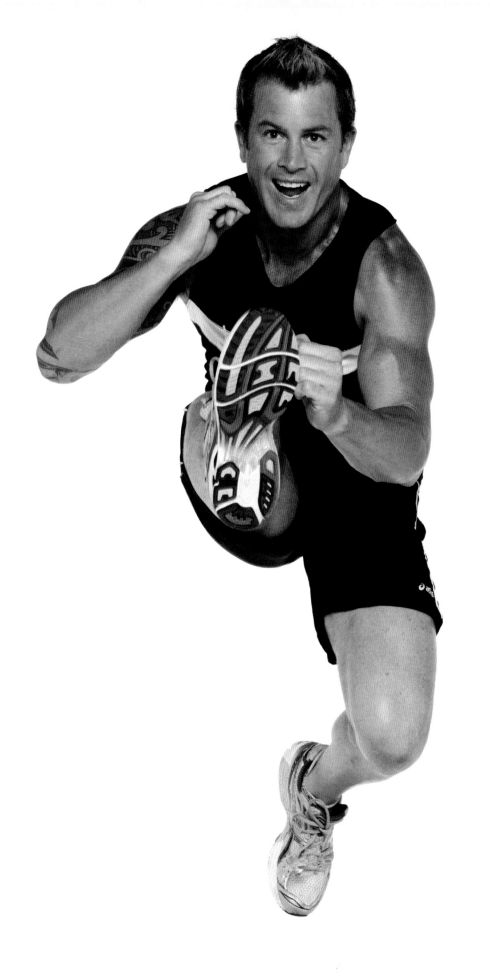

Chapter 12:
Never, ever,
EVER give UP

Your weight-loss journey won't be easy. There will be many a time when you're faced with temptation, when your willpower is low, when you're tired and sore and don't feel like getting up to train, when your goal seems so far away from being reached that you feel like you're never going to get there. Above all else, the one thing that is going to get you over the line is a never-give-up attitude.

Never give up, no matter what the odds.

In Series 5 of *The Biggest Loser*, we had the biggest competitor at that time to ever be on the show, Shannon Bourke, who weighed in at 214 kilos. On the first day of the show we had a challenge for the contestants — they had to run/walk/crawl/whatever for 1 kilometre. It didn't matter how they got there, they just had to get there.

At his weight, Shannon wouldn't walk up the shopping aisle with his girlfriend as he was so embarrassed he'd run out of puff. And here on his first day at

Biggest Loser camp he faced the enormous task of walking 1 kilometre. But it was something I knew he could do. He took off, got to 400 metres and he went down on the ground. He didn't pass out, he didn't collapse, he didn't hurt himself — he just lay down. You could see that his mind had given up. He thought to himself, *Here's a way out, if I just lie down they'll let me go*. But it wasn't to be. It took 30 minutes of me encouraging Shannon to get back up, telling him that this was one of those pivotal moments where if you make the right decision you will change the course of your life and future. He went on another 100 metres down the road and laid down again. At this point he cried like a baby. Here was a 24-year-old man who'd transformed himself to a baby state, curled up crying in the foetal position, begging for me to leave him alone. He used every excuse I'd ever heard, but there was no way I was ever going to give in. I knew that his life depended on him getting up then and there. It took about another 30 minutes and with the help of the medic he got back up. He went another 100 metres and went down again, this time on one knee as you would if you were stepping up to an altar. He had me on one arm and the medic on the other and he screamed, 'Oh, I've broken my knee. I can't move.' Both the medic and I knew that there was nothing wrong with his knee. It was just the only thing he could think of to escape. He lay there for another half an hour crying. Finally we got him up again and by the time he reached the finish line it took about two-and-a-half hours. All of the other contestants had well and truly finished, but almost 3 hours later, he made it.

After this 1 kilometre test I knew I had my work cut out for me and assumed that he would be a nightmare to train. I thought of all the things I respect and identify within a man, and how this guy appeared to be the total opposite. In the first two weeks of training, whatever we did, Shannon would give up. One of the sessions involved the contestants holding a heavy rope above their heads. Shannon was the first one to quit and drop his arms. As the weeks progressed he improved a little, but he'd do something that would earn my respect and then in the next training session give up and do something that would make him lose any little respect he'd earned. Any ground he made would quickly be squashed as he reverted to the old habits that got him into a life of pain and misery.

Then, one day, something shifted in him. Prior to the show, he had to have some serious surgery and doctors had ordered him to get down to 180 kilos before they'd operate as they couldn't guarantee he'd survive the surgery without losing weight. Even when faced with this monumental reality and ultimatum he still found it impossible to lose weight.

He was in his early twenties and already felt like a dead man walking. In fact he *knew* he was a dead man walking as he had already been making plans for checking out: he was going to make sure his finances were in order and that his fiancée would be taken care of; he didn't even think he'd get married.

On this day he stood up and told me that he would never let me down again, that he was ready to change his life. My immediate thought was *I've heard all of this before.* Back then, if I could have chosen to drop the weakest link from my team it would've been him. But at that moment, as he stood before me, something in his thinking shifted and from that day everything changed and he went on to lose 90 kilograms and on a week-in, week-out basis I ended up relying on *him* to keep my team above the yellow line.

This experience made me reassess my beliefs because early on in the game, if given the chance, I would've cut him, and he might have never gone on to have such phenomenal success.

I recently went to his wedding and he looked the best I had ever seen him. He and his wife looked every bit the healthy, happy picture of a bride and groom. When he walked down that aisle I got a tear in my eye (or was it an eyelash?).

What I learned through Shannon is no matter how bad or difficult a situation, never, ever give up on yourself or another person.

Even when the odds are stacked against you and your hands are down, never, ever, EVER give up!

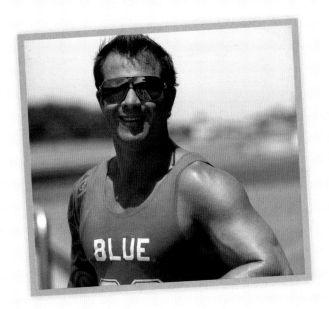

Keep the weight off

Aside from never giving up, what will determine lasting weight-loss success is your ability to pick yourself back up when you fall.

If you have a bad day, don't let it snowball; just get back on track immediately, return to your next healthy meal and workout, and refocus on your goals.

Weight-loss 'mistakes'

Everyone makes mistakes and your weight-loss journey is sure to be fraught with many. It's what you learn from your mistakes that defines you and the results you get.

'If you have a fall

up, get back up a

It's how you reco

it that will defin

pull your socks

l get on with it.

er and deal with

you.'

_____

Shannan Ponton

In order to minimise mistakes in your weight-loss journey, you must prepare yourself mentally, 'get real', understand you and you alone are capable of facilitating change, and you alone reap the rewards of those changes.

Some common examples of 'mistakes' that cause a fall from the weight-loss wagon are:

- Not believing in yourself; when self-doubt surfaces, the wheels fall off.

- Being too comfortable. If you become too comfortable in a relationship or life situation, old habits can start to creep back in.

- Becoming complacent and taking your health, fitness and life for granted.

- Failing to prepare and plan both nutrition and training.

- Quitting before you genuinely have to.

- Still blaming others — my boss increased my workload, my partner keeps junk food in the house, and so on.

- Still hiding behind excuses.

- Clinging on to the victim mentality; refusing to take full responsibility and accountability for changing your habits and life.

- Returning to your old lifestyle: The secret to long-term weight loss is a change in lifestyle. You have to find low-fat, low-calorie, weight-loss friendly foods that you like and are happy to eat as staples for the rest of your life. As soon as you start adding the foods and habits of your old lifestyle, you will regain the weight. The days of your old lifestyle — slack exercise habits, eating anything and everything you want — are done and dusted for good.

- Still thinking and feeling like an obese person. It can take a while for your head to catch up.

- Doing the same workout. If you do the same exercise for long enough your body becomes so used to it that it doesn't have to work nearly as hard as it used to doing the same exercise! Surprising your body by doing varied workouts is essential for avoiding plateaus and keeping the all-important calorie expenditure high.

Power through a plateau

If you've hit a plateau there are three questions to ask yourself.

1. Are you recording all of the calories you're eating?

Make sure you write down *everything* that goes into your mouth and look for unaccounted-for calories you may be missing such as sugar in your tea, bigger portion sizes than you realise you're eating, hidden calories in sauces and dressings. Make sure you really are sticking to your daily calorie quota.

2. Am I doing as much exercise as I believe?

Check your exercise program. Are you really going to the gym three times a week? Are you really exercising for as long as and as much as you think you are? Are you really exercising hard enough?

In order for your body to continually lose weight and change, you must increase intensity, duration or number of workouts per week. For example, if you've been walking 2–3 times a week for 30 minutes and are no longer seeing results, you could: walk for one minute, jog for one minute and repeat for 30 minutes (increase in intensity); walk for 40 minutes (increase in duration); or walk for 4–5 times a week (increase in the number of workouts).

3. Can I be happy at this weight?

If you've hit a plateau that doesn't budge with a shift of gears in your diet and/ or exercise, you may need to reassess your goals. To break through a stubborn plateau will undoubtedly require sacrifice in the form of a lot more exercise and a more stringent diet. You need to work out if it's truly worth the sacrifice. Or maybe you could be happy at this weight?

Tools to keep you on track — diaries, journals, logs and planners

Accountability, honesty and integrity are crucial in sticking with the program. Use logs, journals and diaries to stay true and accountable. Take responsibility for your health, weight, relationships, happiness and place in life — daily!

Weight-loss journal

Simply buy yourself a notebook or diary and make your own weight-loss journal. You can jot down your thoughts about your journey, write your goals, copy inspirational quotes, note your daily weight, record any exercise you did, paste photographs of yourself along the way, and paste inspiring photos of bodies you aspire to (this may even be an old photo of your slimmer, fitter self).

Weigh-in log

Regular weigh-ins are a helpful tool for many as a way of offering instant feedback on your progress. Simply keep a log in a journal, on your computer, or copy and use the sample weigh-in log on page 264, which also has space to keep other body measurements.

Food diary

Often people have calorie amnesia. They conveniently forget the biscuit they had with their tea or the butter they put on the toast. Or people underestimate just how much food and calories they're eating. Seeing it written out in front of you can be a BIG wake-up call. That's why keeping a food diary is critical. You will know exactly how many calories you're putting into your mouth. If you're not losing weight, you've got something tangible to refer to in order to see where you might be going wrong. You may have to adjust your calorie intake, lower it or up your calorie expenditure through more exercise. Losing weight is all about being accountable, and keeping a diet diary is all about accountability for what you eat!

Write everything that goes in! There are no 'no calorie' foods — yes there are calories in the kids' crusts, sugar added to your tea, ice cream off the lid, finishing other people's leftovers, the unplanned biscuit/cake you *had* to eat with friends at afternoon tea. If it goes in the mouth, it goes in the diary!

Copy the sample food diary on page 265 or make a similar template on your computer or in a journal. And remember to add up your total calorie intake each day to make sure you're sticking to your set calorie quota.

Cross-training in the way of incorporating a variety of training modalities, for example, incorporating agility, resistance training, sporting, endurance, impact and non-impact activities is great for optimising results and supercharging your metabolism by keeping your body 'awake'.

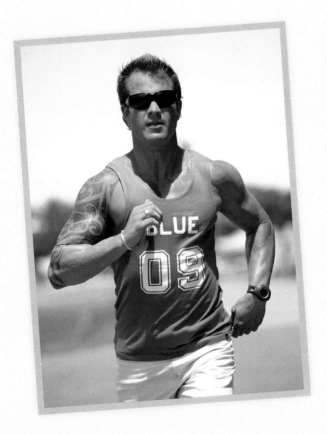

Weigh-in Log

Date	Goals	Weight	Waist	Body fat percentage (optional)	**Additional Girth measurements:**	Chest	Arms	Hips/ buttocks	Mid thigh	Lower leg	**Additional measurements:**								

Food Diary

When photocopying this page, enlarge it so you will have plenty of space to make your entries.

Monday			Tuesday			Wednesday			Thursday			Friday			Saturday			Sunday		
Time	Food ate	Cal	Time	Food ate	Cal	Time	Food ate	Cal	Time	Food ate	Cal	Time	Food ate	Cal	Time	Food ate	Cal	Time	Food ate	Cal
8am	1/2 cup oats	200																		
	Diet yoghurt	84																		
9am	Skim cap	59																		
Daily total:			Daily total:			Daily total:			Daily total:			Daily total:			Daily total:			Daily total:		

NEVER, EVER, EVER GIVE UP

Training diary

The type of training diary you use will depend on the type of training details you want to keep. From the basic ('Went for a 30 minute walk today') to the more technical details such as recording your calorie expenditure, heart rate, time, speed, and distance covered. Keep a basic diary in a weight-loss journal or on your computer, or buy yourself a training diary online or from a sports shop. There are also some great diaries that combine diet intake as well that are called food and exercise diaries.

Resistance training log

It's very motivating to see how much stronger you become over the weeks by recording the weight you lift and how many reps/sets you're able to complete. It also gives you a quick guide to go off each workout so you know what weight you're at, picking up where you left off the workout before. Space is provided in the charts in the 4-phase resistance program in Part 3, use this Resistance Training Log as a spare or for designing your own resistance programs.

Cardio log

Just as it's motivating to see how much stronger you're getting, it's also inspiring to see how much fitter you're getting. Use the log on page 268 to record the results of your cardio sessions. Write down the level or resistance you achieved when using cardio machines or the time it takes, the distance you completed, the heart rate (HR) reached, calories expended (cal), and the speed you reached. When you do your next workout try to better your results — increase the level or speed, go for longer or faster, push your heart rate higher, or aim to burn more calories.

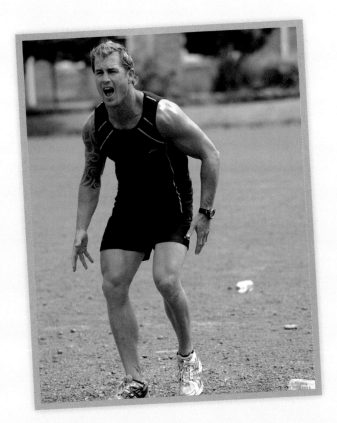

Resistance training log

Name:

Program type/phase:

Resistance training	Date	Set 1	Set 2	Set 3	Set 4	Set 1	Set 2	Set 3	Set 4	Set 1	Set 2	Set 3	Set 4	Set 1	Set 2	Set 3	Set 4	Set 1	Set 2	Set 3	Set 4

NEVER, EVER, EVER GIVE UP

Cardio training log

Date	Level/time	Distance/speed	HR/Cal
1. Tread mill			
2. Cross trainer			
3. Stepper			
4. Outdoor run or walk			
5. Spin or class or circuit			
6. Rower			
7. Cardio of your choice			

Live it up

The best part about losing weight and boosting your energy is that you'll be able to live a better life. No longer will you have to say 'no' to life — 'No son, I can't climb that tree with you,' 'No, I don't feel up to going to a party', 'No I can't buy clothes from that shop', 'No, I'm not fit enough to join the soccer team', 'No, I can't go on holidays because I don't fit in the airplane seat', 'No, I don't want to have sex because I'm too ashamed of my body', 'No, I can't wear sneakers because I can't tie my shoelaces'. Just think of all the things you're missing out on because of your weight?

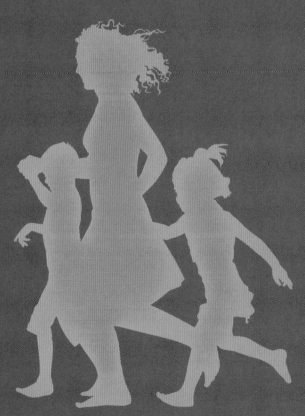

You're going to get your life back! Keep the things you will now be able to do and the life you'll be able to lead firmly in the forefront of your mind at all times of your weight-loss journey. You'll be able to:

- Go clothes shopping wherever you want.

- Run and play with your kids.

- Wear a swimming costume; take a holiday to the beach.

- Walk up a flight of stairs without huffing and puffing.

- Have a social life.

- Find or reconnect with loved ones.

- And much, much more.

Visualise the life you're working towards on a daily basis. See it, feel it, taste it, live it and soon it will become a reality. (Through determination, commitment and discomfort of course. No such thing as a free lunch!)

Final word: Wrap UP

You're going to learn so much about yourself on your weight-loss journey. Before you begin this incredible climb I'd like to leave you with some important life lessons I've picked up along my own journey, which will hopefully help you in yours.

Don't sweat the small stuff

One of the biggest lessons I've learned on *The Biggest Loser* came from one of my contestants on my first season (series 2) with the show, Jules Condon. She was an unassuming lady, quiet in nature, but always in control and nothing ever seemed to get her down or bum her out. But at the same time she was never really as alive as the other contestants were.

It took me about 6 weeks to get to know Jules and to earn her trust. One day I said to her, 'Jules, you're always positive, and I love that about you but it seems like you're not taking the time to smell the roses. What's happened in your life to numb you in this way?' She sat me down on the grass and explained to me what had happened in her life.

As a teenager, her brother Gavin, the closest person in the world to her, suicided and she was devastated. But a few years later, she picked herself up from this tragic time, and went on to marry Tim, who was a childhood friend. Things were looking up.

Facing parenthood was very exciting. She had all of the standard prenatal tests done and everything looked fine. When she gave birth, Jules knew straight away that something was wrong by the look on her mother's face. Jules' mother is a midwife and attended the birth as a support person. The baby was born with Down Syndrome. Jules' husband immediately said, 'I don't care, he's my boy.' And they fell totally in love with Gavin, who is named after Jules' brother.

Jules and Tim's second son Corey was born perfectly healthy and well. A couple of days after Corey's birth, Gavin was diagnosed with leukaemia. Here she is with two kids under the age of two, and Gavin born with Down Syndrome and a diagnosis of leukaemia.

From a scientific point of view, if they had taken the stem cells from the placenta of Corey, born just days before, this potentially could have contributed to lifesaving treatment for Gavin. Without a suitable bone marrow match within the family, they were at the mercy of a national and international bone marrow donor bank, in the event Gavin required a bone-marrow transplant.

Forever positive, Jules went on to talk with doctors about the best ways to help her son, who is now in remission. She discovered there were avenues through in vitro fertilisation to conceive a child to match Gavin's genetic make-up and therefore be a possible bone marrow match.

Even after all this bad luck, Jules and Tim still decided to stay strong and positive and place faith in nature. After all, they thought they still had plenty of time. A third child and possibly a fourth was always planned. Jules went on to conceive and hoped that as a bonus her third child would be a bone marrow match for Gavin. Three months into her pregnancy her husband died of an aneurism.

It was a devastating blow. Two kids (plus one on the way), a sick child and no husband. Still, she focused on her beautiful children and went on to give birth to a perfect, healthy, happy girl called Amy whose stem cells were collected at birth and turned out to be a perfect match for Gavin.

We sat on that lawn for an hour and it was the first and only time I let (had no chance of stopping) the tears roll on camera. And Jules somehow managed to put a positive slant on her life. She said, 'Shannan, I believe that my husband gave his life, so Gavin could have life.'

After such bad luck she still looked at the blessings in her life. She still believed in the bigger picture and that the events in her life were geared towards goodness. She *still* (amazingly!) believed in the greater good of life; that the 'life force' that's there for all of us to share was positive and she could still tap into it and enjoy its fruits.

Her positive outlook really humbled me. Even after 15 years in the fitness and weight-loss industry at that stage, and thinking I'd seen it all, it really made me stop and reassess how I was living my life.

The lesson I took from all of this was don't sweat the small stuff. Because no matter how bad you think you've got it, if you wake up in the morning and you've lost the keys to your car and your three-year-old flushes your iPhone down the toilet, there's nothing to worry about. No matter what happens in life there's always someone who's gone through the same as, or worse than, you. More importantly, there's always someone worse off than you who is more thankful than you.

Life is not a dress rehearsal

My dad had a heart attack a few years back. It was about three in the morning, he was fit and had never been overweight, but a blocked artery from a flap of skin (just bad plumbing!) caused his attack. It wasn't anything that could've been prevented by addressing lifestyle factors; it was just a freak incident. In the ambulance he looked up and said, 'I'm having a heart attack aren't I?' And the ambo said, 'I won't lie to you: yes you are.' And Dad's reply, in his typical philosophical tone, was 'Jesus, I over budgeted mate!' In facing death, he had a moment of clarity: he had plenty of money put away and thought he had the time to enjoy it. Luckily he made it. And at 60 he retired, and he and Mum are now living the best life that they always planned, the life they almost didn't get to live.

We don't get a second go at life. So make time for those things in your life that you dream of achieving and doing — starting today!

When you wake up each morning think about how great your life is and treasure every moment.

At the end of the day when you're lying in a pine box looking up, you've got to be able to look inside your soul, when no one else is around, and ask yourself were you truly happy? Did I live a full, complete life? Do I have any regrets?

And if you don't lose weight, get healthy and take control of your life, you can guarantee, that when all is said and done, you will regret it.

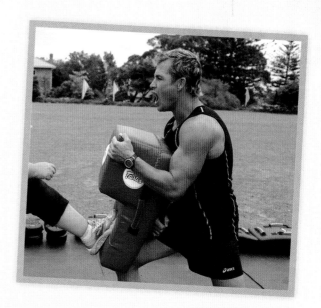

HarperCollins*Publishers*

First published in Australia in 2012
by HarperCollins*Publishers* Australia Pty Limited
ABN 36 009 913 517
harpercollins.com.au

HarperCollins*Publishers*

Level 13, 201 Elizabeth Street,
Sydney NSW 2000, Australia
31 View Road, Glenfield, Auckland 0627, New Zealand
A 53, Sector 57, Noida, UP, India
77–85 Fulham Palace Road,
London W6 8JB, United Kingdom
2 Bloor Street East, 20th floor,
Toronto, Ontario M4W 1A8, Canada
10 East 53rd Street, New York NY 10022, USA

National Library of Australia
Cataloguing-in-Publication entry:

Ponton, Shannan.
    Hard'n up / Shannan Ponton ; Donna Jones.
    ISBN: 9780732292119 (pbk.)
    Reducing diets.
    Weight loss.
    Exercise.
    Physical fitness.
    Jones, Donna, 1978-
613.25

Cover design by Xou Creative, www.xou.com.au
Cover image by Nicholas Wilson
Internal design by Xou Creative
Typeset in Vitesse by Xou Creative
Colour reproduction by Graphic Print Group, Adelaide
Printed and bound in China by RR Donnelley on
128gsm matt art

Image credits: Peter Drew Bevan for photo on page
iii; Stuart Bryce for photos on pages vii, 33, 129, 145,
223, 224, 229, 235, 249, 257, 263, 273; Jason Ierace
for photos on pages 241, 252; Glovebox Sportswear for
photo on page 153; and Nicholas Wilson for photos on
pages vii, 11, 49, 73, 176, 192–221, 253.